ANIMAL HEALTH TECHNOLOGY
Thompson Rivers University
Faculty of Science
P.O. BOX 3010
KAMLOOPS, BRITISH COLUMBIA
CANADA   V2C 5N3

$2007 - \$66.65$

Morgan · Doval · Samii

Radiographic Techniques
The Dog

Joe P. Morgan · John Doval · Valerie Samii

Radiographic Techniques
The Dog

Joe P. Morgan, D.V.M., Vet. med. dr., DACVR
Emeritus Professor

John Doval, Senior Artist

Valerie Samii, D.V.M., DACVR
Lecturer

Department of Surgical and Radiological Sciences,
School of Veterinary Medicine,
University of California, Davis, California

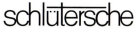

1. English Edition 1998
1. German Edition 1998

© 1998 Schlütersche GmbH & Co. KG, Verlag und Druckerei, Hans-Böckler-Allee 7, D-30173 Hannover.

U. S. A. and Canada: PO Box 30, Williston, VT 05495-0030, Toll free number 888-880-0328

ISBN 3-87706-524-4

Printed by Schlütersche GmbH & Co. KG, Verlag und Druckerei, Hannover

Table of Contents

Preface

This book was written to facilitate the making of radiographic studies of the dog. The underlying concept is to discuss all of the noncontrast views that are to be included for each radiographic study. Included is a review of most common reasons for making the study and special problems relative to the study. A brief written description is made of the positioning and central beam direction for each view. This is enhanced by drawings of both patient positioning and the expected radiograph. Radiographic examinations of the head and spine receive special attention because of the difficulty in radiographic diagnosis of these areas and the requirement for multiple views. The pelvis and hip joints are also the focus for concentration because of the frequency of traumatic injury to this area and because of the frequent requirement for analysis for congenital hip dysplasia. The book strives to provide the student in veterinary medicine as well as the technician working in a busy clinic with helpful suggestions. The book is of greatest value when available during radiographic studies. While the book serves as a convenient reference in the busy practice, it also can be used in teaching.

Davis, October 1997   Joe P. Morgan

Introduction

The radiographic examination

The information obtained in performing a radiographic examination is influenced to a great degree by the manner in which the examination is conducted. A stifle joint examination in a young patient with expected chronic joint disease is usually performed without risk to the dog and the technician or veterinary nurse is free to select from different methods of restraint including both chemical and physical forms. In contrast, the traumatized dog with a fractured femur is more difficult to examine when it also has a pneumothorax and pulmonary contusion. In other words, modification in the use of radiography is often required depending on the condition of the patient. Thus, each patient presents a different challenge to the technician on how to perform the radiographic examination best and most safely and still obtain a diagnostic study. It is our intent to describe what we feel to be the positioning that will result in the production of a diagnostic radiographic study. It would be a serious error to believe that there is a single method that is appropriate for a particular radiographic study in all patients. For this reason, we have described frequently in the following pages different methods for positioning and restraint. Particular methods that are valuable for use in one dog may be contraindicated because of unique injury or disease in another dog. It is hoped that the reader will use the information contained in the following pages as a guide and will develop additional methods that serve well in their clinic.

Patient preparation

Preparation of the patient is divided into two areas: preparation of the "outside" of the patient, including the skin and haircoat; and the "inside" of the patient, including consideration of the contents of the gastrointestinal and urogenital systems. Many "nonvisualized" objects can interfere with the quality of the radiographic image in addition to those objects that are easily seen.

Preparation of the outside of the patient includes an examination of the skin and haircoat. Removal of collars and restraining devices is necessary in cervical and thoracic studies. A wet haircoat causes prominent film artifacts because the hair sticks together to form a radiopaque object. Some contrast agents that are clear may look like water on the skin, but because they have a high content of iodine will cause radiopaque film artifacts. A quick brushing of the haircoat can result in the identification of foreign bodies such as plant material, dirt, or gravel. External splints and casts can make evaluation of underlying anatomical structures difficult and often a different positioning is required. It is recommended that all external support devices be removed prior to radiographic evaluation when possible. In some patients, the splints or casts may need to remain in position. In preparing a limb for radiography, it may be necessary to stabilize an injured limb so that it can be moved without the risk of further injury to the soft tissues around a suspected fracture. A dog with a suspected spinal fracture should be strapped to a support board so that the dog can be moved for radiography without risking further injury to the spinal cord.

Preparation of the patient's internal organs must also be considered. A stomach full of liquid/ingesta crowds other abdominal organs and makes their evaluation difficult. A small bowel full of bone chips and other debris causes radiopaque shadows that makes evaluation of the abdomen almost impossible. Fecal material can cause shadows as dense as some bones and its removal enhances eva-luation of the intrapelvic structures. The amount of urine within the bladder determines how easily that organ is identified on the radiograph. However, distension of the bladder crowds other caudal abdominal organs, making their identification more difficult or impossible.

Certain conditions affect radiographic quality but are often not appreciated until after examination of the original study. Some of these can be controlled, while others cannot. These conditions include the presence of air or fluid within the body cavities. The presence of pleural fluid creates a tissue density that may prevent an underlying lung lesion from being seen on the radiograph. Preparation for radiography of that dog might include drainage of the pleural effusion prior to radiography. The value of ultrasonography must be appreciated in patients such as this.

Patient restraint

Patient restraint includes both chemical and physical forms. The selection is usually dependent on: (1) the medical status of the patient, (2) the radiographic examination to be performed, (3) the nature of the dog, and (4) the wishes of the owner. Consideration of all of these points determines the choice of immobilization. Some hospitals have a policy that excludes technicians from being in the examination room during a radiographic study while others rely on tight collimation of the primary X-ray beam and the use of lead shields, aprons and gloves that enables technicians to assist directly in positioning and get to remain shielded and outside the primary beam.

Chemical restraint may include sedation or anesthesia. Positioning a patient that is deeply sedated or anesthetized is definitely easier than handling a dog that is fully awake. The study can be performed more quickly, and yields a higher quality radiograph. It is often difficult to convince technicians and veterinarians that the time used in chemically sedating the patient is quickly recovered by the speed in which the radiographic study can be performed in the sedated or

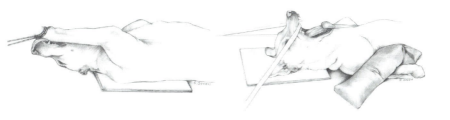

anesthetized patient. In the event of chemical restraint, it is recommended that the dog be intubated. However, the presence of an endotrachial tube may compromise some studies and its location needs to be considered. For clarity, the endotracheal tube has not been included in the drawings in this book.

Methods of physical restraint include the use of: (1) tie-down devices, (2) sandbags, (3) compression bands, or (4) the gloved hand. While many different forms are illustrated in this manual, the manner of use of these restraints is limited only by the imagination of the technician. Tie-down devices may be made of line, bungee cord, or gauze. Generally they are attached to the dog's limb using a half-hitch type of knot and are stretched and attached to the table edge or tube stand, wrapped around a sandbag layed on the table top, or tied to a sandbag that is hung over the edge of table. Gauze is frequently used in smaller patients and is especially valuable in radiography of the head and mouth.

Sandbags are extremely important in positioning for radiography because of the quickness with which they can be used. They are available in various sizes and shapes appropriate for the size of the patient and the body part to be radiographed and can be placed over a limb or body part or can be wrapped around a limb. It is important to keep the sandbags clean or within a bag that can be cleaned, to prevent film artifacts.

Tape is available in various forms but is not conveniently used as a restraint device because of the dirt and debris that adheres to it. It is possible to use and discard it after using once.

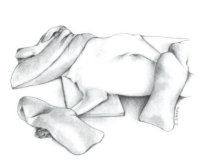 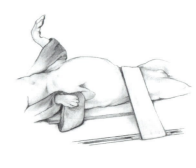

Use of a compression band across the thorax or abdomen is a less commonly used technique of physical restraint because many X-ray tables do not have a convenient method or device for attaching the band. Devices originally fabricated for use with the table often have a ratchet that permits tightening of the band quickly and easily. In the absence of a table built for use with a compression band, it is possible to tie sandbags to the ends of a cloth or canvas strip and

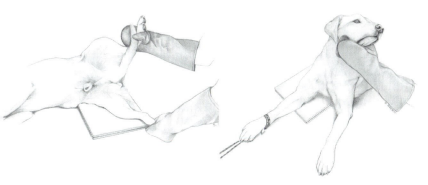

place the band across the patient with the sandbags hanging over the edges of the table. The weight of the sandbags can be varied in consideration of the size of the dog.

The use of the gloved hand as a restraint device needs to be included because there are patients in which the use of chemical restraints or other forms of physical restraint are contraindicated. Each individual reading this manual must determine how often gloved hands are to be used in radiographic studies. The gloved hand should never be used so it is positioned within the primary X-ray field. This means that the character of the collimator and the size of the primary X-ray beam need to be well understood. Also, use of a gloved hand as a restraint device implies that the assistant is within the room and his or her body must then be protected by some form of shielding device or apron.

Throughout this manual, various restraint devices/techniques are illustrated. These are by no means the only methods that may be utilized for a particular examination. For clarity, some devices may be omitted from diagrams.

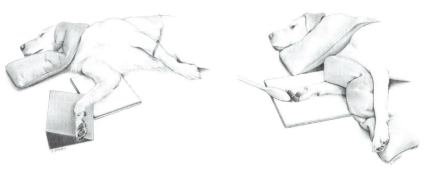

Whenever a restraining device is placed within the primary beam, it must be one that can be cleaned regularly. This is important because of transmission of disease and because of the adherence of radiopaque material to the device that creates film artifacts. Sand-bags are often placed within a washable cover. Tie-down ropes can be replaced frequently and tape and gauze used only once.

Patient positioning devices

Patient positioning devices are used to place a body part into a particular position prior to radiographic examination and ensure stability of the part to be examined. The positioning device may in addition: (1) cause rotation of a body part, creating obliquity, (2) elevate an affected body part from the table top, or (3) remove an unaffected body part from the beam. They may assume the form of: (1) a wedge or block-shaped sponge, (2) a trough, (3) a sandbag, (4) plastic or wooden spoons, or (5) a tie-down device. The use of gauze or tape rolls in radiography of the mouth and teeth is a common practice; however, these devices cannot be cleaned and should not be used more than once.

If the positioning device is used within the primary X-ray beam, it must be radiolucent. This is the reason that sponges, purchased from an X-ray supply company, are used so commonly in radio-graphy of the dog. If the positioning device is to be used outside the beam, it may be radiopaque. This dictates how and in what circum-stances sandbags can be used in positioning.

Troughs are made from wood, plastic, or sponge material. The construction determines whether they can be placed within the primary beam. Positioning devices should be washable to avoid creation of film artifacts due to dirt and contrast medium. Washable covers may be purchased for sponges and sandbags. Tie-down devices need to be replaced frequently, and tape and gauze used only on one patient.

Oblique views

Oblique views of the dog are generally accomplished by repositioning the patient relative to the primary X-ray beam. This means that the X-ray tube remains in position, with the vertical beam perpendicular to the table top. Oblique views are made in this manner because the position of the patient can usually be altered more easily and more quickly than the position of the X-ray tube. However, in some instances, it is necessary to position the patient in a relatively standard manner and angle the X-ray tube so that the beam strikes the patient at a predetermined angle to the table top. The extreme example of this form of repositioning is used with a patient in which the tube is lowered to a level with the table top and turned through 90° so that the primary beam is horizontal.

Cassette positioning devices

If using a horizontal X-ray beam, it is necessary to hold the cassette in a vertical manner. This may be accomplished through use of a wall-mounted device, especially in radio-graphy of the thorax or abdomen. In radiography of the ex-tremities, the cassette is usually rested on the table top, and sandbags or a special holder are used to maintain its position. These special cassette hol-ders attach to the table top through suction cups or to the edge of the table top by tightening "jaws". Some cassette holders may be shifted in position through the use of pivotable "arms".

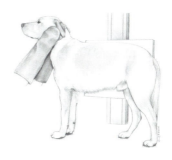

Method of beam identification

In this book, terminology is used to identify the passage of the X-ray beam through the body. The first term describes the body surface first contacted by the X-ray beam and the second term is used to describe that body surface from which the X-ray beam exits. Thus a beam might be dorsoventral (DV) or ventrodorsal (VD) in orienta-tion. Oblique and special views are more difficult to label and are described more specifically. If the beam enters dorsally and laterally and exits ventrally and medially, it is a DLat/VMed oblique beam. Most X-ray beams are directed vertically to the longitudinal axis of the part radiographed. If the beam is angled to this axis, it may be described as $x°$ cranial or caudal, or rostral or caudal, or proximal or distal. The point of centering of the beam further describes the passage of the X-ray beam along with its relationship to the table top. It may be possible to state that the X-ray beam is within a plane within the body. Knowledge of the planes of intersection through the body are of additional value in understanding tube and body positioning. Thus, the beam may pass in a craniocaudal direction (entering the body part on the cranial surface and exiting on the caudal surface), be centered at the site of a particular anatomical part, pass through the sagittal plane of the body part, and be perpendicular to the table top.

Film label

A method is necessary by which the image on the radiograph is identified so that it is possible to determine which body part was radiographed, the manner in which the patient was positioned, and the direction of the X-ray beam. In radiography of the head, thorax, abdomen, pelvis, and spine always use a right marker (R) to indicate laterality. On all lateral views, the marker should identify the side of the body that is dependent, i.e. the side that is underneath. On oblique views, use both R and left (L) markers to assist in determining how the oblique view was made. When radiographing a part of a limb in craniocaudal or dorsopalmar/plantar orientation, place the R or L marker on the lateral side.

Patient measurement

Measurement of the patient is necessary to determine the appropriate machine settings, the radiographic technique or "X-ray technique", to be used, based on chart specifications. Comments are included within the descriptions of certain views suggesting the best manner in which to take these measurements and extrapolate the appropriate exposure factors from the chart.

Identification of film

In addition to a label that identifies the body part and how the patient was positioned, it is necessary to identify the film as to the date it was made, patient and client name, and name of the clinic or hospital where taken. Different types of film markers are available for this purpose with some much easier to use than others. All are satisfactory if used correctly.

Type of X-ray machine

It is not the purpose of this manual to describe the X-ray machine and explain how it functions. However, comments are made within the descriptions of the views if the nature of the machine may present a limitation in how the method may be utilized. An important feature in the discussion of horizontal beam radiography is whether the tube stand permits lowering of the tube and turning it on its axis. Oblique views may require that the tube be able to turn within its holder.

Grid

Certain methods use a film cassette placed on the table top just under the part to be radiographed. Radiography of thicker body parts may require use of an under-table tray that holds the film cassette as well as a grid. The grid may be movable or stationary. The drawings showing patient positioning in this book have the cassettes drawn on the table top, or in a vertical holder for horizontal views, so the reader can easily determine their location. Placement of the cassette into a tray beneath the table is determined by patient size. Comments are included as to when a grid is required and are usually based on the thickness of the part radiographed; however, certain exceptions exist. The thorax, being filled with air, does not require use of a grid in some larger dogs. Grids are usually used to decrease secondary radiation when radiographing:

>11 cm abdomen, pelvis, proximal limbs, head

>15 cm thorax.

Focal-film distance

An altered focal-film distance is mentioned in certain special views and represents the distance from the X-ray tube to the film. This distance is decreased in certain studies, especially in dental radiography.

Screen versus nonscreen systems

Screen systems or nonscreen films can both be used in veterinary radiography. Most clinics prefer not to deal with the additional exposure chart required for a nonscreen system. In some studies, in which the dog is anesthetized, movement is not a problem, and a nonscreen film produces an image of much greater quality, their use should be encouraged. Screen film systems are produced with marked variations in speed and it is important that these speeds be known. Some clinics will choose to use a faster system for thoracic, abdominal, spinal, and pelvic studies, while using a slower system for studies of extremities and the head.

Thorax

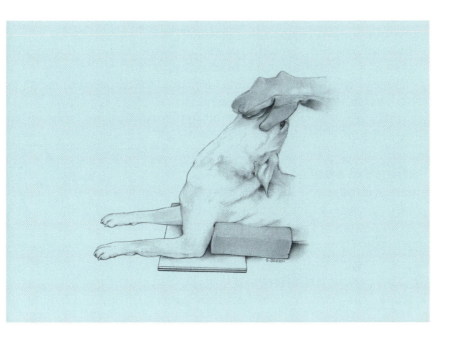

Thorax

Introduction
- a most important radiographic study because it permits evaluation of several body systems
- used for detection of congenital, traumatic, inflammatory, neoplastic, and degenerative lesions
- most valuable for detection of disease of the lungs, cardiovascular system, mediastinum, and thoracic wall
- value in comparison of ventrodorsal and dorsoventral views as well as right lateral and left lateral views
- studies should be made in all patients prior to surgery or institution of any lengthy therapy

Patient preparation
- remove collar or lead rope
- inspect haircoat for matted hair, debris, or foreign bodies
- note amount of body fat and adjust the radiographic technique accordingly

Sedation or anesthesia
- study can be made with the patient awake, sedated, or anesthetized
- chemical restraint is not required and usually is contraindicated if pulmonary or cardiac disease is suspected

Views
- recommended views
    - lateral (vertical beam)
    - dorsoventral (vertical beam)
    - ventrodorsal (vertical beam)
- special views
    - thoracic inlet (skyline view)
    - oblique views from VD or DV position (vertical beam)
    - lateral (horizontal beam)
        in sternal recumbency
        in dorsal recumbency

in standing position on four feet
in erect position on hindfeet
– ventrodorsal (horizontal beam)
in lateral recumbency
standing erect on hindfeet

X-ray technique
– increase 10 kVp (or increase kVp by 15%)
  – with pleural fluid
  – with infiltrative lung disease
  – in obese patient
– decrease 10 kVp (or decrease kVp by 15%)
  – with pleural air
  – in thin patient

Inspiration versus expiration
– attempt to make study at full inspiration to evaluate pulmonary disease
– expiration study is of value for the identification of minimal pleural air

Use of grid
– > 15 cm measurement
– use grid in smaller dogs with suspected pleural fluid, infiltrative lung disease, or with obesity

Comments
– dogs that have been in prolonged lateral recumbency due to anesthesia or morbidity often have atelectasis of the dependent lung, which compromises filling of the lung lobes with air and makes adequate evaluation of the dependent lobes difficult radiographically because of the increased tissue density
– do not succumb to the temptation of taking only a single lateral view for the study of the thorax since pulmonary lesions as well as pleural air or fluid may be missed on a single view
– in markedly deep-chested breeds, such as the sight hounds, two DV/VD projections of the thorax are taken at different exposures to evaluate cardiac and pulmonary structures adequately

Thorax – lateral view (vertical beam)

Body
– place in lateral recumbency with vertebral and sternal columns parallel to the table surface
– place wedge sponge under sternum
– use compression band across abdomen for restraint

Forelimbs
– extend limbs cranially so elbows are over manubrium
– place sandbags across forelimbs or use tie-down rope

Hindlimbs
– extend limbs caudally
– place sandbags across hindlimbs or use tie-down rope

Head and neck
– extend head in natural position
– place sandbag across neck

X-ray beam centering
– direct vertical beam to 5th rib interspace
– center in the transverse plane just caudal to the body of the scapula

Collimation
– include thoracic inlet and diaphragm

Comments

- select same lateral recumbent view (right or left) for all studies to become familar with radiographic appearance of organs as seen with that positioning
- if location of thoracic wall or pleural lesion is known, position that side nearest to table top for best radiographic detail
- if location of pulmonary lesion is known, position that side uppermost for best radiographic detail
- the image of a discrete lesion may be magnified by positioning the lesion away from the table top
- free pleural fluid shifts downwards, causing "silhouetting" of the adjacent organs
- in dogs with pleural fluid this positioning causes fluid to move to a dependent position and encourages inflation of the upper lung field

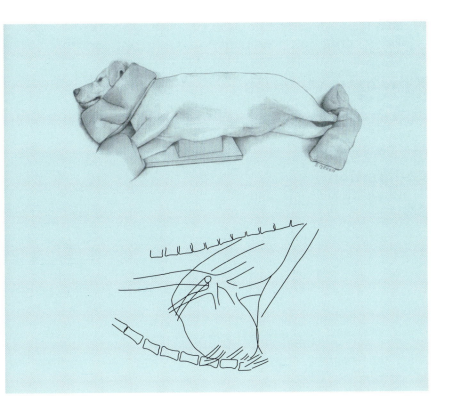

Thorax – dorsoventral view (vertical beam)

Body
- place in sternal recumbency
- use sponge trough or place sandbags lateral to abdomen

Forelimbs
- extend limbs cranially with limbs abducted
- place sandbags across forelimbs or use tie-down rope

Hindlimbs
- flex into frog-leg position
- place sandbags across hindlimbs

Head and neck
- extend head in natural position
- place sandbag over dorsum of neck

X-ray beam centering
- direct vertical beam to 5th rib interspace
- center in the transverse plane just caudal to the body of the scapulae

Collimation
- include thoracic inlet and diaphragm

Comments

- view of choice for evaluation of cardiac silhouette size and shape
- can place sandbags lateral to elbows to force forelimbs into adduction to displace scapulae laterally so they are not superimposed over cranial thoracic lung field
- in dogs with pleural fluid this positioning causes fluid to move to a dependent position and encourages inflation of the upper lung field

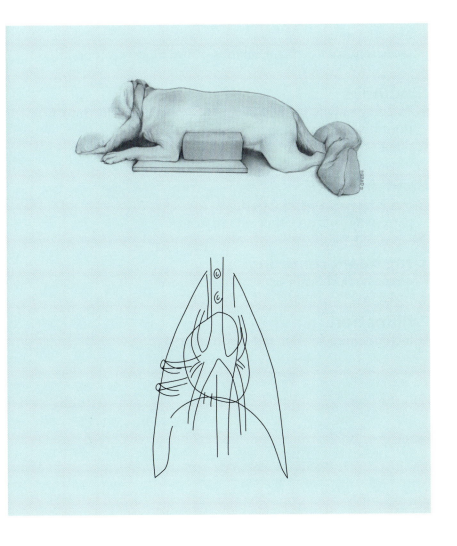

Thorax – ventrodorsal view (vertical beam)

Body
- place in dorsal recumbency
- use sponge trough or place sandbags lateral to abdomen
- place compression band across caudal abdomen
- palpate sternum and position on midline

Forelimbs
- extend cranially
- place sandbags across forelimbs or use tie-down rope

Hindlimbs
- extend caudally in fully extended position or flex into frog-leg position
- place sandbags across hindlimbs or use tie-down rope

Head and neck
- extend head in neutral position
- place sandbags on either side of head

X-ray beam centering
- direct vertical beam on xyphoid process

Collimation
- include thoracic inlet and diaphragm

Comments

- view often used in dogs with painful hip joint disease that resent DV positioning, since frog-leg positioning is less painful
- view of choice in dogs with pleural effusion to position fluid in the paraspinal gutters allowing better evaluation of the cardiac silhouette
- view usually used in dogs in which it is difficult to control positioning
- may position sandbags lateral to abdomen to prevent rotation
- may be necessary to use gloved hands on limbs to achieve good positioning

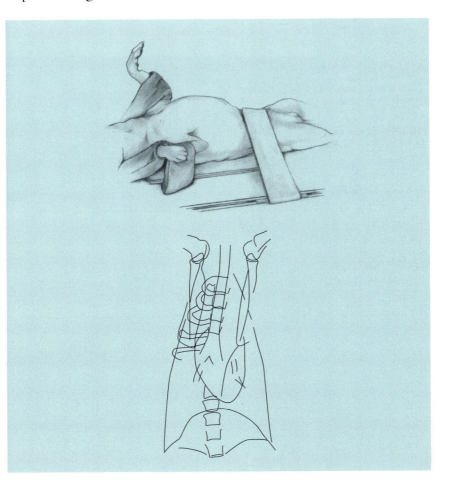

Thorax – thoracic inlet (dorsocranio – ventrocaudal oblique)

Body
- place in ventral recumbency
- use sponge trough
- place compression band across back
- palpate manubrium process and position on midline

Forelimbs
- extend cranially with limbs abducted
- place sandbags across forelimbs or use tie-down rope

Hindlimbs
- flex into frog-leg position

Head and neck
- hyperextend head with tie-down rope or use gloved hand

X-ray beam centering
- direct 30° dorsocranio-ventrocaudal angled beam on manubrium process

Collimation
- include thoracic inlet

Comments

- view used to evaluate tracheal size, shape, and position at thoracic inlet
- use 40" (100 cm) tube-film distance
- decrease thoracic radiographic technique by 10 kVp (or 15%)
- use table-top method regardless of patient size
- often referred to as "skyline view"

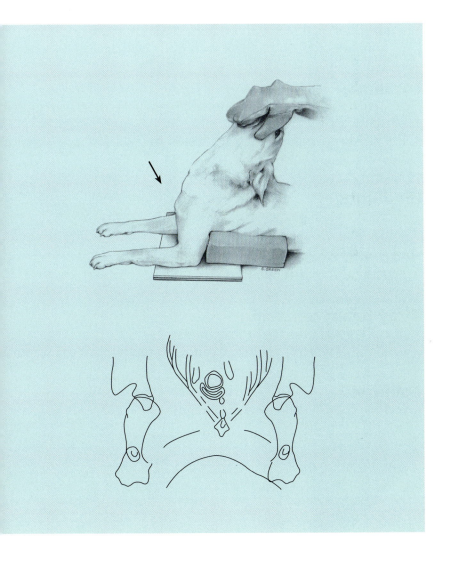

Thorax – lateral view (horizontal beam)

Body
- study can be made with the dog placed in several positions
  - in sternal recumbency with either right or left side against cassette
  - in dorsal recumbency with either right or left side against cassette
  - standing on 4 feet with body held against cassette
  - standing erect on hindfeet with body held against cassette

Forelimbs
- try to extend forelimbs to remove elbows from thoracic region in all views
- use tie-down ropes or gloved hands to hold forefeet (requirement varies with position)

Hindlimbs
- extend caudally (varies with position)

Head and neck
- extend head in natural position

X-ray beam centering
- direct vertical beam to 5th rib interspace
- center in transverse plane just caudal to the body of the scapulae

Collimation
- include thoracic inlet and diaphragm

Comments

- use wall-mounted or table-mounted cassette holder to position cassette or use sandbags to hold cassette vertical on table top
- use sponge block to elevate the body if necessary to permit centering on cassette
- recumbent views made in dorsal or ventral recumbency permit fluid to move downward and pleural air to move upward
- standing view on four feet permits fluid to move dependently around the sternum and pleural air to move dorsally
- erect standing view on hindfeet permits fluid to move dependently around the diaphragm and pleural air to move dorsally into the cranial thorax
- wait several minutes after positioning patient for fluid and air to relocate before making exposure
- contraindications for these studies include any positioning that results in a pressure from loculated or trapped pleural fluid or an intrathoracic mass that compresses existing inflated lung

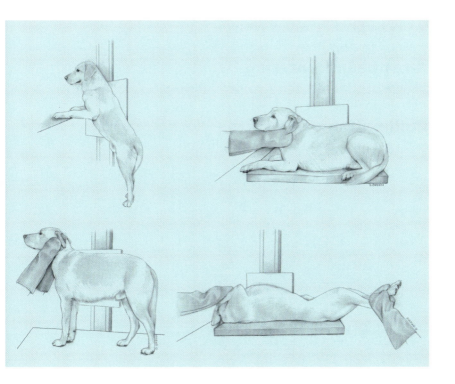

Thorax – ventrodorsal view (horizontal beam)

Body
– study can be made with the dog
  – in lateral recumbency with back against cassette
  – standing erect on hindfeet

Forelimbs
– pull limbs cranially
– use tie-down ropes or gloved hands

Hindlimbs
– extend caudally

Head and neck
– extend head in natural position

X-ray beam centering
– direct vertical beam on xyphoid process

Collimation
– include thoracic inlet and diaphragm

Comments

- need some type of cassette holder to position cassette or use sandbags to hold cassette vertical on table top
- if necessary use sponge block to elevate the body to permit centering on cassette
- recumbent ventrodorsal view permits pleural fluid to move downward to one side and pleural air to move dorsally to the other side
- standing erect on hindfeet permits pleural fluid to move dependently around the diaphragm and the pleural air to move dorsally to the cranial portion of the thorax
- wait several minutes for fluid and air to reposition before making exposure
- in the standing erect view, it is easiest to have two persons each stand lateral to the dog and hold it erect using gloved hands
- if looking for evidence of free abdominal air, positioning on the left side is recommended, so air within the fundus does not interfere with identification of free abdominal air.

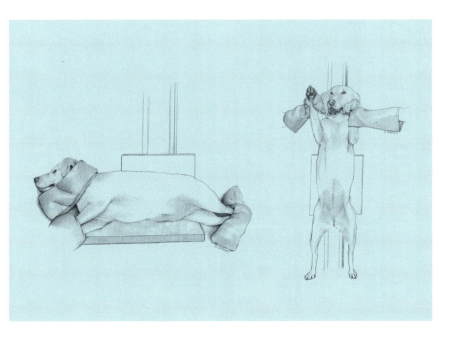

Notes

Abdomen

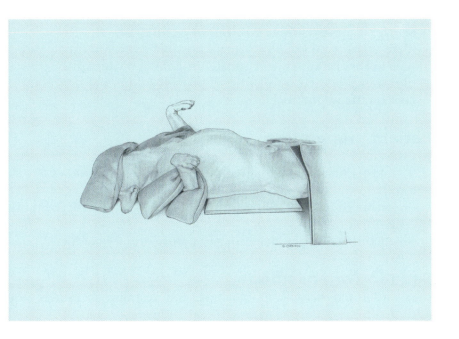

Abdomen

Introduction
- more difficult to visualize abdominal structures because of the presence of tightly compressed fluid-density organs
- possible to create contrast studies by use of air, barium sulfate suspensions, and iodinated contrast agents
- many studies are used to evaluate possible gastrointestinal lesions while others are used to evaluate urogenital problems
- ultrasound is used frequently to provide additional information concerning abdominal lesions

Patient preparation
- external
    - inspect haircoat for matted hair, debris, foreign bodies
- internal
    - withhold feed for 12 hours prior to study if possible to empty gastrointestinal system
    - encourage dog to defecate and empty urinary bladder

Sedation or anesthesia
- not required because positioning and restraint is usually not difficult
- study can be made with patient awake, sedated, or anesthetized

Views
- recommended views
    - lateral (vertical beam)
    - lateral for male urethra (vertical beam)
    - ventrodorsal (vertical beam)
    - dorsoventral view (vertical beam)
- special views
    - lateral (horizontal beam)
        in sternal recumbency
        in dorsal recumbency
        in standing position on four feet
        in erect position on hindfeet

- ventrodorsal (horizontal beam)
  in lateral recumbency
  in erect position on hindfeet

X-ray technique
- increase kVp if suspect peritoneal fluid

Use of grid
- use grid if measurement is >11 cm

Special techniques
- use of compression paddle to shift overlying gas or fecal-filled bowel loops
- use of injected rectal air to identify location of rectum (pneumocolon)
- use of swallowed gastric air to identify location of stomach (negative gastrogram)

Inspiration *versus* expiration
- make study in expiration to permit cranial positioning of the diaphragm and maximum separation of abdominal organs

Comments
- with colon full of feces consider use of enema or wait for defecation
- with stomach full of ingesta consider use of emetic or wait for normal emptying
- with full urinary bladder take the dog for a walk or catheterize
- peritoneal fluid causes decrease in serosal detail and alternative imaging (ultrasonography) should be considered for adequate evaluation
- increase technique and use cone-down views for better evaluation of spinal, pelvic, or femoral lesions that have been noted on abdominal study
- presence of abdominal fat enhances diagnostic quality of study, making a radiograph of a "fat cat" most diagnostic

Abdomen – lateral view (vertical beam)

Body
- place in right lateral recumbency
- use compression band across thorax
- the spine and pelvis are often studied on the lateral view, so use a sponge wedge beneath sternum to position the body more accurately

Forelimbs
- extend limbs cranially
- place sandbags across forelimbs or use tie-down rope

Hindlimbs
- extend caudally but avoid marked extension as this tightens the abdominal wall compressing abdominal organs
- place sponge between femurs to improve lateral position
- place sandbags across hindlimbs or use tie-down rope

Head and neck
- extend head in natural position
- place sandbag across neck

X-ray beam centering
- if large dog
  - center on last rib for study of stomach and liver
  - center on midabdomen for bladder, uterus, or prostate
- if small or medium-sized dog
  - direct beam just caudal to the last rib for entire abdomen

Collimation
- include both diaphragm and pelvis if possible

Comments

– measure body size at level of last rib to determine radiographic technique
– use right lateral view
  – to cause fundus of stomach to be filled with air
  – to cause descending colon to be filled with air
– use left lateral view
  – to cause pyloric antrum and duodenum to be filled with air
  – to cause cecum and ascending colon to be filled with air

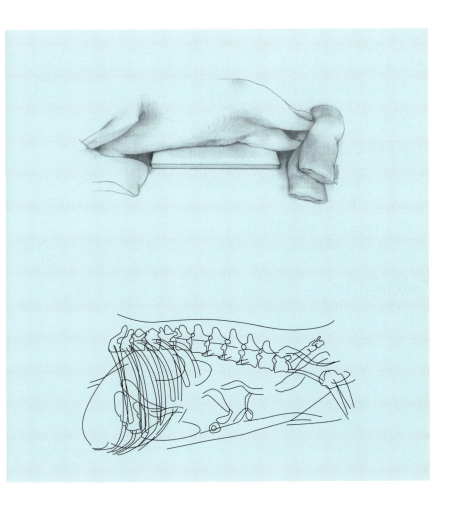

Abdomen – lateral view for male urethra (vertical beam)

Body
– place in right lateral recumbency
– use compression band across thorax
– place a sandbag to position tail

Head and neck
– extend head in natural position
– place sandbag across neck

Forelimbs
– extend limbs cranially
– place sandbags across limbs or use tie-down ropes

Hindlimbs
– flex to maximum position
– place sandbags across limbs or use tie-down ropes

X-ray beam centering
– direct vertical beam on ischium

Collimation
– include caudal abdomen and pelvis

Comments

- measure at level of acetabulum
- decrease radiographic technique for soft tissue study
- use low kVp to create a high contrast radiograph to permit easier visualization of calculi
- use table-top positioning regardless of patient size
- include os penis in study
- avoid superimposition of femurs over urethra

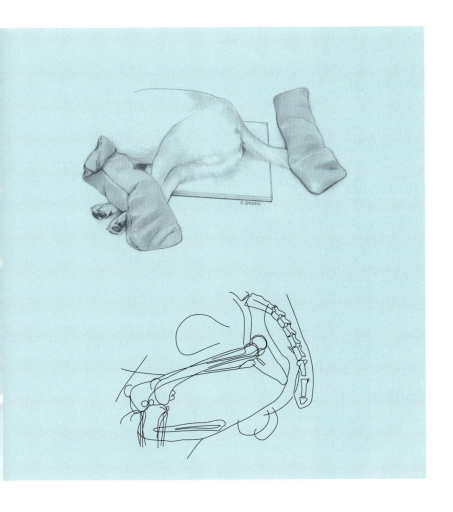

Abdomen – ventrodorsal view (vertical beam)

Body
- place in dorsal recumbency
- place in trough
- palpate xyphoid process on midline to insure correct body position

Forelimbs
- extend limbs cranially
- place sandbags across forelimbs or use tie-down rope or hold feet with gloved hands

Hindlimbs
- extend caudally or flex into frog-leg position
- avoid marked extension since this tightens the abdominal wall
- place sandbags across hindlimbs or use tie-down ropes or compression band or hold feet with gloved hands

Head and neck
- extend head in natural position
- place sandbags on either side of head or use compression band or hold head with gloved hands

X-ray beam centering
- if large dog
  - center on last rib for study of stomach and liver
  - center on midabdomen for bladder, uterus, or prostate
- if small dog
  - direct beam just caudal to the last rib for entire abdomen

Collimation
- include both diaphragm and pelvis if possible

Comments

- measure at level of last rib to determine radiographic technique
- use ventrodorsal position in smaller dogs that are resistent to positioning in sternal recumbency
- ventrodorsal positioning places air in pyloric antrum and duodenum and descending colon

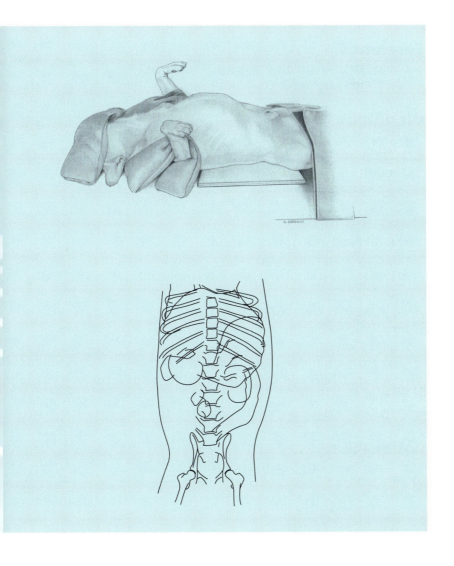

Abdomen – dorsoventral view (vertical beam)

Body
– place in sternal recumbency
– place in trough
– palpate spinous processes on midline to ensure correct body position

Forelimbs
– extend cranially with elbows placed laterally
– place sandbags across forelimbs

Hindlimbs
– partially extend caudally or place in frog-leg position
– avoid positioning limbs so that weight is on patellas since this is painful
– place sandbags across hindlimbs or use gloved hands

Head and neck
– extend head in natural position
– place sandbags on either side of head
– may need to use gloved hands to support head in awake dog

X-ray beam centering
– direct vertical beam just caudal to last rib
– if large dog center
    – on last rib for study of stomach and liver
    – on midabdomen for study of bladder or uterus or prostate
– if small dog center
    – on last rib for entire abdomen

Collimation
– include both diaphragm and pelvis if possible

Comments

- positioning allows the abdominal viscera to "fall" into a more normal position for radiography
- insure that spine is straight and on line with sternum
- dorsoventral position is more successfully used in larger dogs
- dorsoventral positioning places air in gastric fundus and transverse colon
- kVp may need to be increased by 10 (or 10-15%) above what is normally used for ventrodorsal techniques

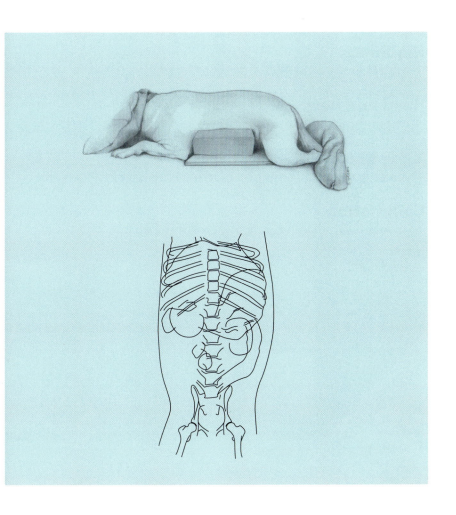

Abdomen – lateral view (horizontal beam)

Body
– study can be made with the dog in several positions
  – in sternal recumbency with side against cassette
  – in dorsal recumbency with side against cassette
  – standing on four feet with body held against cassette
  – standing erect on hindfeet with body held against cassette

Forelimbs
– extend limbs cranially (as directed by position)

Hindlimbs
– extend limbs caudally (as directed by position)

Head and neck
– extend head in natural position

X-ray beam centering
– direct horizontal beam just caudal to the last rib

Collimation
– include both diaphragm and pelvis if possible

Comments
– use cassette holder to position cassette or use sandbags to hold cassette vertically on table top
– use sponge pad to elevate the body if necessary
– measure at level of last rib
– these views permit movement
  – of free peritoneal air upwards
  – of free abdominal fluid downwards
  – of air and fluid within hollow viscera permitting identification of stomach or bowel
– wait several minutes after positioning patient for free peritoneal air to relocate before making exposure
– positioning often requires use of gloved hands
– right lateral and left lateral views produce essentially the same radiograph

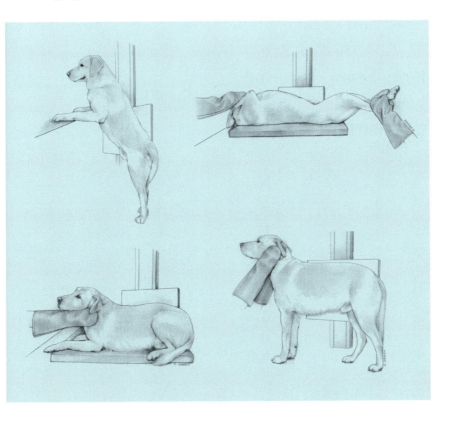

Abdomen – ventrodorsal view (horizontal beam)

Body
– study can be made with the dog standing erect or in lateral recumbency
  – in lateral recumbency with back against cassette
  – standing erect on hindfeet

Forelimbs
– extend limbs cranially (as directed by position)

Hindlimbs
– extend limbs caudally (as directed by position)

Head and neck
– extend head in natural position

X-ray beam centering
– direct horizontal beam just caudal to the last rib

Collimation
– include diaphragm and pelvis

Comments

– use cassette holder to position cassette or sandbags to hold cassette on table top
– use sponge block to elevate the body if necessary
– measure at level of last rib
– these views permit movement
    – of free peritoneal air upwards
    – of free abdominal fluid downwards
    – of air and fluid within hollow viscera permitting identification of stomach or bowel
– the standing positioning often requires use of two people each standing lateral to the dog using gloved hands
– wait several minutes after positioning patient for free peritoneal air to relocate before making exposure
– if looking for evidence of free abdominal air, left lateral dependent positioning is recommended, so air within the fundus does not interfere with identification of free abdominal air

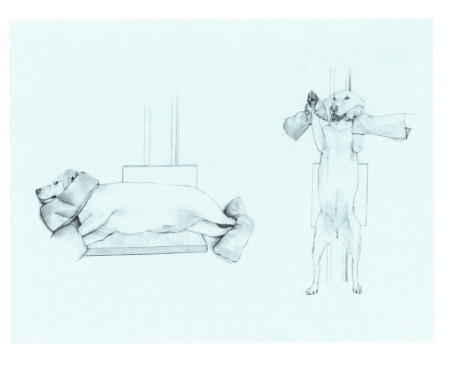

Notes

Head

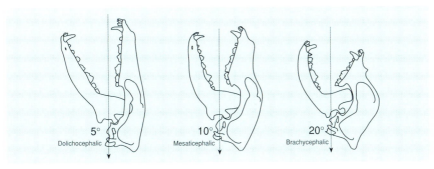

5° Dolichocephalic   10° Mesaticephalic   20° Brachycephalic

Head

Introduction
- the most difficult body region to evaluate radiographically because of difficulties in positioning and wide variation in appearance of anatomical structures
- because of the unique morphology many special views are used in radiographic evaluation
- limitation of study to dorsoventral and lateral views provides little information not determined by physical examination
- studies have little, if any, value in examination of intracranial lesions
- CT has become useful in more specifically defining inflammatory, traumatic, and neoplastic lesions
- the following are considered separately within the text:
    - nasal region, paranasal sinuses, maxillary region
    - mandible
    - dental studies
    - pharyngeal studies
- the maxilla, bullae, and temporomandibular joints are considered within studies of the head

Patient preparation
- remove collar and lead rope
- inspect hair coat for matted hair, debris, foreign bodies
- consider whether endotracheal tube need be removed during film exposure
- identify position of ears to insure they are not folded under the head where they create prominent radographic shadows
- consider position of tongue since it causes a prominent soft tissue shadow
- position of the body is important since it has an influence on how the head is positioned

Sedation or anesthesia
- not required for a routine survey study
- heavy sedation is required in many patients

– anesthesia is required for special views and is strongly recommended for all views if possible

Views
– recommended views – with vertical beam
  – lateral
  – ventrodorsal
  – dorsoventral
– special views
  – oblique views for maxilla
  – frontal view
  – fronto-occipital view for occipital bone
  – fronto-occipital view for foramen magnum
  – open-mouth view for tympanic bullae
  – lateral oblique view for temporomandibular joints
  – lateral oblique view for tympanic bullae

X-ray technique
– measure nose for studies of nasal passages and sinuses
– measure further caudal for studies of the calvarium
– consider use of nonscreen film for open-mouth and dental studies

Use of grid
– not usually required for studies of the head except in very large breeds

Comments
– determination of proper positioning is made most difficult when considering the various sizes and shapes of dog's heads
– all views are not of value in all breeds
– there are problems in understanding the use of each view
– use of the different views creates difficulties in interpreting the anatomical structures
– every view is not indicated in each clinical situation
– generally it is best to make more views than thought necessary while the patient is under sedation or anesthesia, rather than having to return for additional studies at a later time

Head – lateral view

Body
– place in lateral recumbency with affected side next to table top
– compression band across thorax or abdomen

Forelimbs
– place limbs in a neutral position
– place sandbag across forelimbs or use tie-down rope

Hindlimbs
– place limbs in a neutral position
– place sandbag across hindlimbs or use tie-down rope

Head and neck
– place cassette on table top
– position head on cassette
– extend head in natural position
– place a sponge wedge beneath the mandible
– position so the interpupillary line is perpendicular to the table top
– position so the midsagittal line is parallel to the table top
– place pinnae of ears dorsally (especially note the lower ear)
– place a sandbag against the dorsum of the head so the dog cannot move its head into a hyperextended position
– endotracheal tube can remain in position

X-ray beam centering
– direct vertical beam along interpupillary line

Collimation
– include incisor teeth and first cervical segments

Comments
- can use pinnae as "handles" to assist in positioning head in awake patient
- use of a carpenter's level device placed along the length of the nose is often helpful in insuring the head is parallel to the table
- use spoon or paddle to assist in controlling position of head
- mouth can be closed or open for this study

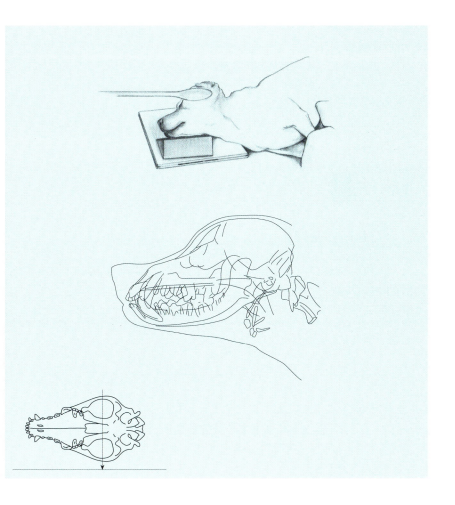

Head – dorsoventral view

Body
- place in sternal recumbency using a trough
- use a compression band across thorax or abdomen or position sandbags lateral to dog's body to maintain good dorsoventral position

Forelimbs
- place limbs in a neutral position
- place sandbag across forelimbs or use tie-down rope

Hindlimbs
- place limbs in a neutral position

Head and neck
- place cassette on table top
- position head on cassette
- extend head in natural position
- place pinnae of ears laterally
- place sandbag against the dorsum of neck
- endotracheal tube can be removed or remain in position

X-ray beam centering
- direct vertical beam on interpupillary line

Collimation
- include incisor teeth and first cervical segments

Comments
- the shape of the mandible naturally positions the head for the dorsoventral view
- insure the interpupillary line is parallel to the table top
- can use pinnae as "handles" to assist in positioning head in awake patient
- an alternative method of positioning is provided by making the patient more comfortable by elevating the head from the table top by resting it on a large sponge block

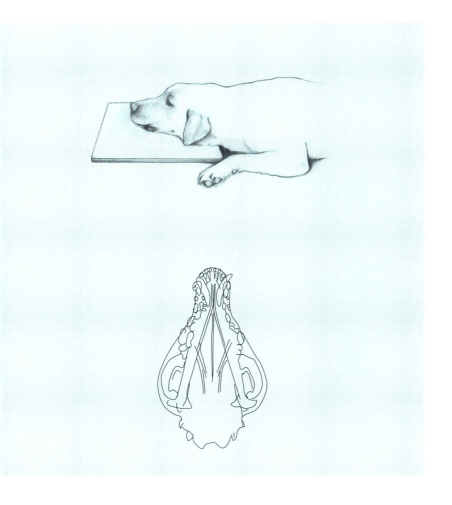

Head – ventrodorsal view

Body
– place in dorsal recumbency using a trough
– position sternum on midline
– use a compression band across thorax or abdomen or position sandbags lateral to the body to maintain good ventrodorsal position

Forelimbs
– place limbs in a neutral position
– place sandbag across forelimbs or use tie-down rope

Hindlimbs
– place limbs in a neutral position
– place sandbag across hindlimbs or use tie-down rope

Head and neck
– place cassette on table top
– position head on cassette
– place head in natural position
– place small sponge block under nose
– pull nose toward table top until horizontal rami of mandible are parallel to table top
  – hold nose in position with paddle or spoon
  – use compression band across mandible
  – use tie-down rope
– place pinnae of ears laterally
– place sandbags on either side of the head
– endotracheal tube can be removed or remain in position

X-ray beam centering
– direct vertical beam on intermandibular space

Collimation
– include incisor teeth and first cervical segments

Comments

- strive to have the body of the mandible parallel to the table top
- can angle X-ray beam caudal to rostral to project body of the mandible parallel to table top if cannot depress dog's nose
- positioning can be altered by depressing dog's nose so it is closer to the table top
- breeds with short noses are difficult to position for this view and the ventrodorsal view is recommended only in dolichocephalic breeds
- can use pinnae as "handles" to assist in positioning head in awake patient

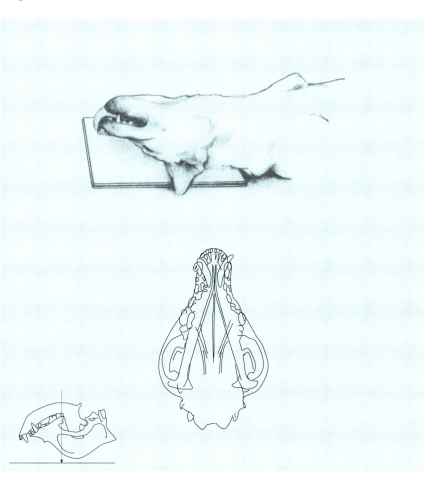

Head – oblique views for maxilla

Body
– place in dorsal recumbency using a trough
– position sternum laterally toward side to be studied
– maintain position by placing a compression band across thorax or abdomen or position sandbags lateral to dog's body

Forelimbs
– place limbs along thoracic wall
– place sandbag across forelimbs or use tie-down rope

Hindlimbs
– place limbs in a neutral position
– place sandbag across hindlimbs or use tie-down rope

Head and neck
– place cassette on table top
– position head on cassette
– use gauze strip or tape to rotate head so that midsagittal plane and the hard palate are at a 45° angle to the table top
– place sponge block under nose
– pull nose toward table top
   – use gauze strip or tape placed behind upper canine teeth
   – tie gauze strip or tape to table or around sandbag
   – hold nose in position with wooden spoon or paddle
– place pinnae of ears laterally
– place sandbags on either side of the head
– endotracheal tube can be removed or remain in position
– open mouth slightly

X-ray beam centering
– direct vertical beam on upper 3rd premolar

Collimation
– include all teeth and paranasal sinuses

Comments
– positioning can be altered by depressing dog's nose
– if cannot change position of the head consider changing the direction of the X-ray beam so it is at a 45° angle
– can use roll of gauze or speculum to open mouth
– breeds with short noses are difficult to position for this study
– usually make both oblique views so results can be compared
– use same exposure as for standard views

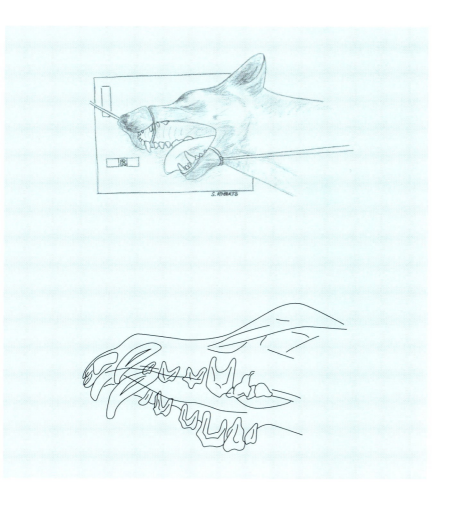

Head – frontal view

Body
- place in dorsal recumbency using a trough
- position sternum on midline
- place compression band across thorax or abdomen or position sandbags lateral to dog's body to maintain ventrodorsal position

Forelimbs
- place forelimbs along side of thorax
- place sandbag across forelimbs or use tie-down rope

Hindlimbs
- place limbs in a neutral frog-leg position
- place sandbag across hindlimbs or use tie-down rope

Head and neck
- place cassette on table top
- position head on cassette
- place head with nose pointing upwards toward tube
- wrap gauze strip or tape around dorsum of nose
    - pull caudally on gauze
    - angle hard palate 10°–20° caudorostrally to table top
    - tie gauze strip or tape to table edge or wrap around sandbag
- place sandbags against both sides of head
- place pinnae of ears laterally
- endotracheal tube can be removed or remain in position

X-ray beam centering
- direct vertical beam between eyes parallel to dorsum of nose

Collimation
- include frontal sinuses

Comments

– positioning can be altered by depressing dog's nose
– this view is extremely difficult, or impossible, to obtain in dogs with "dome-shaped" heads (e.g. Chihuahua)
– breeds with long noses do not have prominent frontal bones, making positioning for this view more difficult
– can use pinnae as "handles" to assist in positioning head
– decrease X-ray technique because of decrease in tissue thickness
– maintain 40" (100 cm) tube-film distance

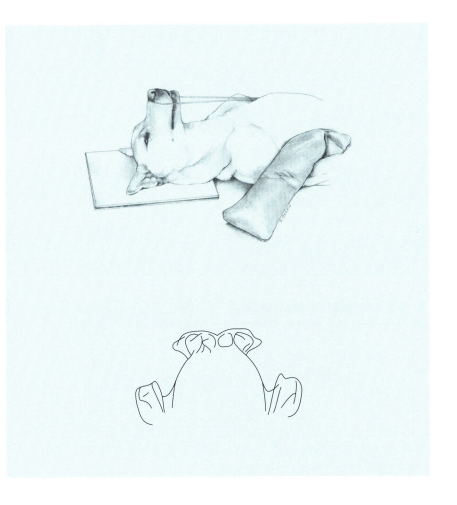

Head – fronto-occipital view for occipital bone and foramen magnum

Body
- place in dorsal recumbency using a trough
- position sternum on midline
- place compression band across thorax or abdomen or position sandbags lateral to dog's body to maintain ventrodorsal position

Forelimbs
- place limbs along side of thorax
- place sandbag across forelimbs or use tie-down rope

Hindlimbs
- place limbs in a neutral frog-leg position

Head and neck
- place cassette on table top
- position head with nose pointing upwards
- wrap gauze strip or tape around dorsum of nose
  - pull nose caudally
  - angle hard palate caudally 30°– 45° to table top
  - tie gauze strip or tape to table edge or wrap around sandbags
- place sandbags against both sides of head
- place pinnae of ears laterally
- endotracheal tube can be removed or remain in position

X-ray beam centering
- direct vertical beam between eyes

Collimation
- include base of skull

Comments

– this view places the occipital bone parallel to the cassette
– the shape of the head in different breeds alters positioning for this view
– can use pinnae as "handles" to assist in positioning head in awake patient
– the difference between this view and the frontal view is that the nose in this view is pulled further caudally
– decrease X-ray technique appropriately
– maintain 40" (100 cm) tube-film distance

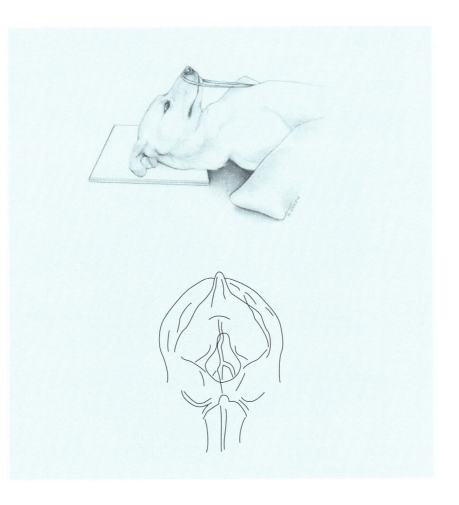

Head – open-mouth view for tympanic bullae, C1, and odontoid process

Body
- place in dorsal recumbency using a trough
- position sternum on midline
- place compression band across thorax or abdomen or position sandbags lateral to dog's body to maintain ventrodorsal position

Forelimbs
- place forelimbs next to thorax
- place sandbag across forelimbs or use tie-down rope

Hindlimbs
- place limbs in a neutral frog-leg position

Head and neck
- place cassette on table top
- position head on cassette
- place head with nose pointing upwards
- wrap gauze strip or tape around nose just caudal to upper canine teeth
    - pull gauze strip or tape rostrally
    - tie gauze strip or tape to side of table cranially and laterally or wrap around sandbags placed cranially and laterally
- wrap gauze strip or tape around lower jaw caudal to lower canine teeth
    - pull gauze strip or tape caudally
    - tie gauze strip or tape caudally to end of table or wrap around a sandbag placed caudally
- pull both gauze or tape strips tightly until mouth opens wide
- adjust position of head so the line that bisects the angle created by the hard palate and the body of the mandible is perpendicular to table top
- place sandbags against both sides of head
- place pinnae of ears laterally
- endotracheal tube removal is strongly recommended

X-ray beam centering
- direct vertical beam to bisect angle created by the hard palate and the body of the mandible

Collimation
– include tympanic bullae, C1, and odontoid process of C2

Comments
– positioning of head for this study is breed-dependent (see drawings below)
– this view is most useful for visualizing the odontoid process and the bullae
– position the head carefully in patients where trauma is suspected
– it is possible to position the head more accurately for this view by adjusting the angle between the hard palate and the central X-ray beam to be
    – 20° in brachycephalic breeds
    – 10° in mesaticephalic breeds
    – 5° in dolichocephalic breeds
– decrease X-ray technique appropriately

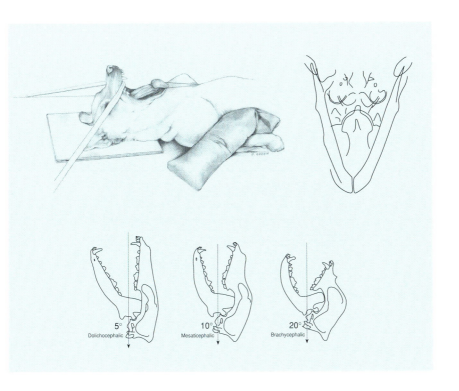

Head – lateral oblique view for temporomandibular joints

Body
- place in lateral recumbency
- place the joint to be studied downwards
- place compression band across thorax or position sandbags next to dog's body to maintain lateral position

Forelimbs
- extend limbs in a neutral position
- place sandbag across forelimbs or use tie-down rope

Hindlimbs
- place limbs in a neutral extended position

Head and neck
- place cassette on table top
- place head on cassette
- rotate dorsum of head toward the table top
- position head so hard palate is at a 10° angle to the table top
- place sponge under mandible to maintain obliquity
- elevate nose so midsaggital plane of head is at the following angle with the table top
    - 25°–30° in brachiocephalic breeds
    - 15° in mesaticephalic breeds
    - 10° in dolichocephalic breeds
- place sponge under nose to maintain elevation and rotation
- place sandbag against top of head
- place pinnae of ears dorsally
- endotracheal tube can be removed or remain in position

X-ray beam centering
- direct vertical beam below eye

Collimation
- include temporomandibular joints

Comments
- may place gauze strip or tape around nose and lower jaw and tie to table top to assist in positioning nose
- note that the head is rolled slightly and the nose is elevated slightly in obtaining this view.
- breed influences positioning (see drawings below)
- the studies can be made with the mouth open or closed
- radiography of both temporomandibular joints recommended so studies can be compared

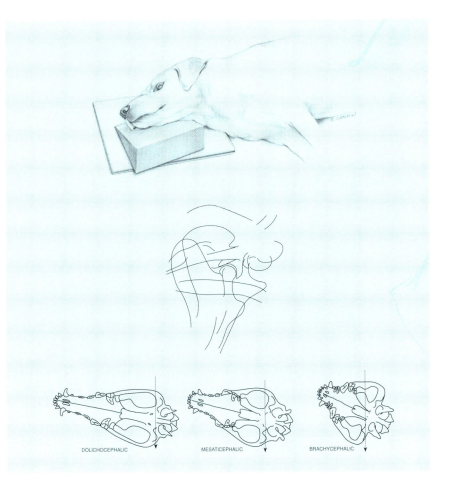

DOLICHOCEPHALIC   MESATICEPHALIC   BRACHYCEPHALIC

Head – lateral oblique view for tympanic bullae

Body
- place in lateral recumbency on side to be studied
- place compression band across thorax or position sandbags next to dog's body to maintain lateral position

Forelimbs
- extend limbs in a neutral position
- place sandbag across forelimbs or use tie-down rope

Hindlimbs
- place limbs in a neutral extended position

Head and neck
- place cassette on table top
- position head on cassette
- place sponge under nose
- place head so midline is parallel with the table top
- rotate dorsum of head 30° toward the table top
- place wedge sponge beneath nose to maintain position
- it is not necessary to open the mouth for this view
- endotracheal tube can be removed or remain in position
- place sandbag against top of head
- place pinnae of ears laterally

X-ray beam centering
- direct vertical beam below eye

Collimation
- include tympanic bullae and temporomandibular joints

Comments

– can place gauze around nose and lower jaw to assist in positioning nose
– can use pinnae as "handles" to assist in positioning head in awake patient
– a radiograph of the opposite tympanic bulla should be made for comparison

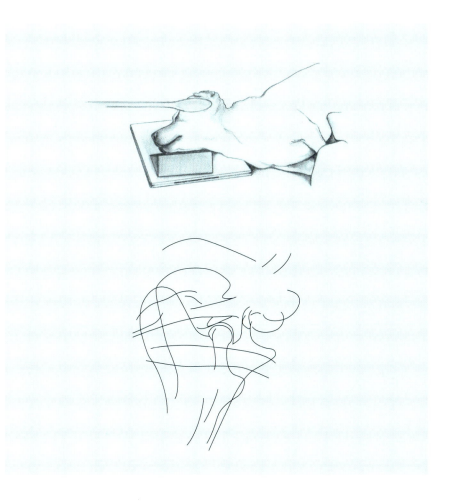

Mandible

Introduction
– problems are associated with proper positioning of the mandible in breeds of various sizes and shapes
– should separate study of the mandible from that of the head
– mandible is usually studied for fractures, osteomyelitis, periodontal disease, dental disease, tumor affecting bone or teeth

Patient preparation
– remove collar and lead rope
– inspect hair coat for matted hair, debris, foreign bodies
– consider whether endotracheal tube need be removed while taking exposures
– evaluate position of tongue since it causes a prominent soft tissue shadow

Sedation or anesthesia
– sedation is required in most instances
– anesthesia is strongly recommended

Views
– recommended views
  – lateral
  – oblique views
– special views
  – oblique views of the temporomandibular joints (p 70)
  – ventrodorsal view with intraoral film (p 76)
  – dorsoventral view of head (p 58)

X-ray technique
– measure nose for technique
– measure further caudal for studies of the body and temporo-mandibular joints
– consider using nonscreen film for open-mouth studies and dental studies

Use of grid
– usually a grid is not required for studies of the head except in the giant breeds

Comments
– difficult to project the lower caudal molars clearly
– DV view of head includes mandible but it is only seen to a limited extent due to superimposition of the bone forming the nasal cavity (p 58)

Mandible – ventrodorsal intraoral view

Body
– place in dorsal recumbency using a trough
– position body so sternum is on midline
– place compression band across thorax or position sandbags lateral to dog's body to maintain ventrodorsal position

Forelimbs
– place limbs beside the thoracic wall
– place sandbag across forelimbs or use tie-down rope

Hindlimbs
– place limbs in a neutral position

Head and neck
– place head on table top
– extend head in natural position
– loop gauze strip or tape caudal to the maxillary canine teeth
    – pull upper jaw so the hard palate is parallel to the table top
    – tie gauze or tape to table edge or wrap around sandbag
– place one corner of non-screen film holder into mouth as far caudally as is possible
– use gauze strip or tape over the rostal portion of the mandible to position the body of the mandible parallel to table top
– place pinnae of ears laterally
– endotracheal tube can be left in position

X-ray beam centering
– direct vertical beam into intermandibular space

Collimation
– include all lower teeth

Comments

– angle the X-ray beam caudorostrally if it is not possible to pull nose toward table top, so palate is parallel to table top
– can use pinnae as "handles" to assist in positioning head
– note the position of the dog's tongue
– position the non-screen film gently to avoid penetration by the teeth of the paper cover on the film
– this view permits excellent evaluation of the rostral portion of the mandible
– maintain a 40" (100 cm) tube-film distance
– decrease the exposure appropriately

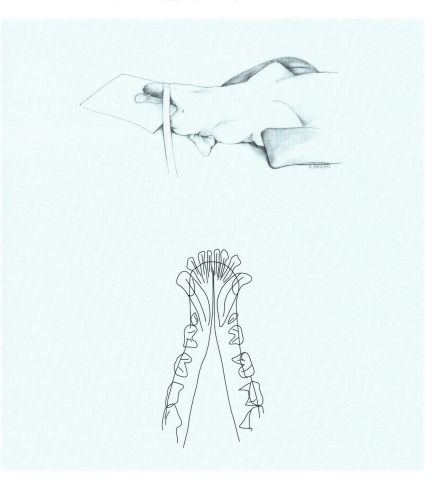

Mandible – oblique view

Body
– place in sternal recumbency using a trough
– position body so sternum is shifted laterally away from half of mandible to be studied
– place compression band across thorax or position sandbags lateral to dog's body to maintain dorsoventral position

Forelimbs
– place limbs in a flexed position
– place sandbag across forelimbs or use tie-down rope

Hindlimbs
– place limbs in a neutral position

Head and neck
– place cassette on table top
– place head on cassette
– extend head in natural position
– rotate dorsum of head to an angle of 30° with the table top
– place gauze roll or speculum between either pair of canine teeth
– open mouth as far as is possible
– use sponge wedge to elevate mandible so the body of the lower half of the mandible is parallel to the table top
– place pinnae of ears laterally
– endotracheal tube can be left in position
– pull tongue laterally away from the half of the mandible to be studied

X-ray beam centering
– direct vertical beam into mouth centering on the 3rd lower premolar

Collimation
– include all lower teeth and body of mandible

Comments

- it is recommended that radiographs of both halves of the mandible are made
- breed type determines the length of the body of the mandible and predicts the success in making this view
- a shorter jaw is difficult to position parallel to the table top
- can use pinnae as "handles" to assist in positioning head
- remember that a metallic speculum creates a radiopaque shadow on the radiograph

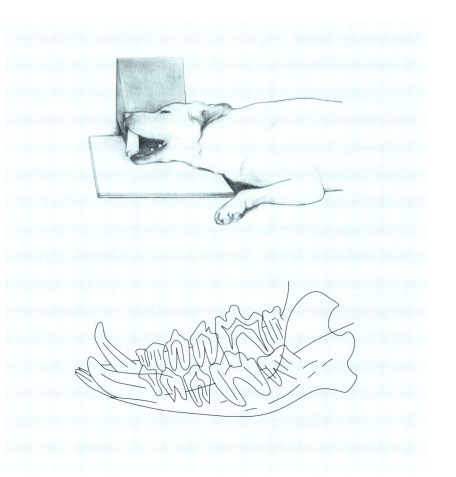

Nasal Passages, Paranasal Sinuses, and Maxillary Region

Introduction
- a commonly used study following a history of intractable epistaxis that is nonresponsive to therapy
- of value in study for suspected intranasal foreign body or tumor
- of value in the determination of extent of injury in trauma patients
- radiograph is most informative in long-nosed breed dogs

Patient preparation
- remove collar and lead rope
- inspect haircoat for matted hair, debris, foreign bodies
- consider whether endotracheal tube need be removed during exposure
- identify position of pinnae of ears to insure they are not folded under the head
- consider position of tongue since it causes a soft tissue shadow

Sedation or anesthesia
- heavy sedation is required in most patients
- anesthesia is strongly recommended to obtain most definitive open-mouth studies

Views
- recommended views
  - lateral
  - open-mouth ventrodorsal
  - open-mouth dorsoventral (intraoral)
- special views
  - dorsoventral or ventrodorsal view of the entire head are of little value in study of the nasal cavity because of overlying shadows of the tongue and mandible (p 58, 60)
  - oblique lateral views as described in studies of the head are of value in studies of the nasal cavity (p 62)

– frontal view is important since nasal disease often extends into the frontal sinuses (p 64)

X-ray technique
– measure nose for studies of nasal passages and sinuses
– measure further caudal for studies of the calvarium
– consider use of nonscreen film for open-mouth and dental studies

Use of grid
– a grid is not required for studies of the nasal region

Comments
– certain views are used for an emergency study while additional views are used for specific patients
– study has particular value in determining selection of biopsy site
– since most lesions have an inflammatory component in addition to the basic lesion, it is possible for the result of a biopsy to be misleading
– radiographs are most easily evaluated by making a comparison of one side with the other side
– CT scans of the nasal cavity better characterize and differentiate inflammation from neoplasia than radiography

Nasal study – ventrodorsal open-mouth view

Body
– place in dorsal recumbency using a trough
– position body so sternum is on midline
– position a compression band across thorax or position sandbags lateral to dog's body to maintain ventrodorsal position

Forelimbs
– place limbs beside the thoracic wall
– place sandbag across forelimbs or use tie-down rope

Hindlimbs
– place limbs in a neutral position

Head and neck
– place cassette on table top
– place head on casette
– extend head in natural position
– loop gauze strip or tape just caudal to the lower canine teeth
  – include the tongue and endotracheal tube (if present) within gauze or tape
  – pull mouth open
  – tie gauze strip or tape to foot of table or wrap around a sandbag
– loop gauze or tape loop just caudal to the upper canine teeth
  – tie gauze strip or tape to edge of table top
  – position upper jaw so hard palate is nearly parallel to tabletop
– place pinnae of ears laterally
– place sandbags laterally
– endotracheal tube can be repositioned laterally

X-ray beam centering
– angle beam rostrocaudally 20° to 30° to the table top
– center the beam on the hard palate
– beam should be near parallel to the body of the mandible

Collimation
– include all of nasal cavity as far caudally as is possible

Comments
– length of nose determines the quality of the radiograph obtained
– in short-nosed dogs it is difficult to open the mouth wide enough to make this view
– can use pinnae as "handles" to assist in positioning head
– use a 40" (100 cm) tube-film distance
– decrease X-ray technique appropriately

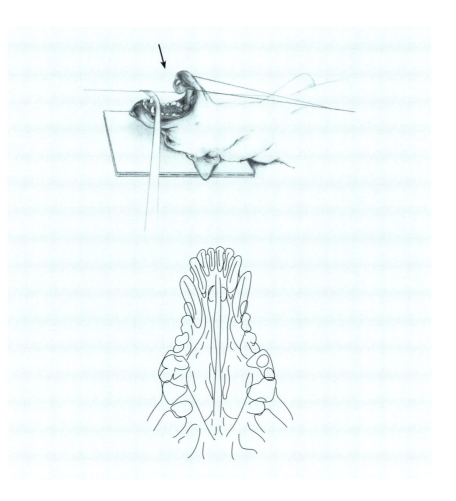

Nasal study – dorsoventral intraoral view

Body
- place in sternal recumbency using a trough
- position body so sternum is on midline
- place compression band across thorax or position sandbags lateral to dog's body to maintain dorsoventral position

Forelimbs
- place limbs in an extended abducted position
- place sandbag across forelimbs

Hindlimbs
- place limbs in a frog-leg flexed position

Head and neck
- place head on table top
- extend head in natural position
- open the mouth and place a corner of a non-sceen film as far caudally into the mouth as possible
- close mouth gently, since teeth striking the film can cause a pressure artifact or may even cut the paper film holder
- tongue and endotracheal tube are beneath the film
- place pinnae of ears laterally
- place sandbags lateral to head

X-ray beam centering
- angle beam 10° to 15° rostrocaudally to the table top
- center beam on the midline just rostral to the eyes

Collimation
- include all of nasal cavity as far caudally as is possible
- the caudal portion of the nasal cavity is usually not included on the film because of the limitation in film positioning

Comments
- length of nose determines the quality of the radiograph obtained
- in short-nosed dogs it is difficult to position the film caudally
- can use pinnae as "handles" to assist in positioning head
- it is possible to use a thin screened cassette for this study, however it cannot be positioned as far into the mouth because of its thickness
- this is an excellent study to view the upper incisor teeth
- maintain a 40" (100 cm) tube-film distance whether using a screen or non-screen technique
- decrease X-ray technique appropriately

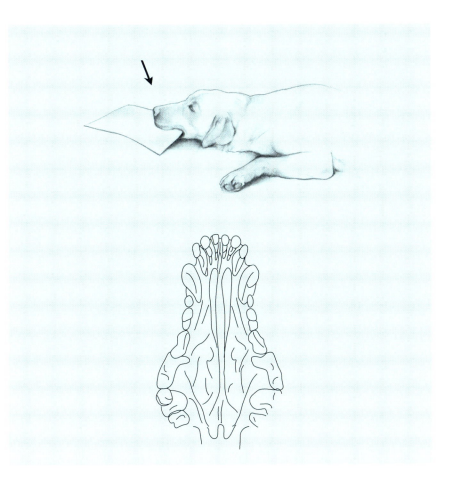

Dental Studies

Introduction
- the studies may be made following trauma or may be a study suggested because of suspected dental or periodontal disease
- teeth are frequently affected by dental or periodontal tumors
- oblique views as described for the maxilla and mandible can serve as part of the dental studies (p 62–79)
- other studies may be made by positioning the X-ray film intraorally
- problems in radiography of the teeth are often due to variants in size and shape of the head

Patient preparation
- consider whether the endotracheal tube is within the radiation field
- identify position of ears to insure they are not folded under the head
- consider position of tongue since it causes a prominent soft tissue shadow

Anesthesia
- anesthesia required for most studies

Views
- recommended views
  - oblique views
- special views
  - intraoral film for ventrodorsal view of mandibular incisors
  - intraoral film for dorsoventral view of maxillary incisors
  - intraoral film for oblique view of mandibular incisors
  - intraoral film for oblique view of maxillary incisors

X-ray technique
- nonscreen film for intra-oral studies
- decrease tube-film distance for nonscreen film studies to 30" (75 cm)
- decrease exposure factors for screen technique
- select higher machine settings for non-sceen technique

Use of grid
- a grid is not required for dental studies

Comments
- oblique views of the head and mandible provide an opportunity to study the premolars and molars
- special views are necesssary to study the incisors or canine teeth
- use of intraorally positioned dental film produces higher quality radiographs than use of extraorally positioned screened casssette technique
- potential problems in radiation safety exist with use of intraoral film because of the higher radiation exposures required to achieve high detail nonscreen radiographs if the technician is within the examination room during the exposure

Dental studies – oblique view of upper premolars and molars

Body
- place in dorsal recumbency using a trough
- position sternum laterally toward side to be studied
- place compression band across thorax or abdomen or position sandbags lateral to the dog's body to maintain ventrodorsal position

Forelimbs
- place limbs in a neutral position
- place sandbag across forelimbs

Hindlimbs
- place limbs in a neutral position

Head and neck
- place cassette on table top
- place head on cassette
- place sponge block under nose
- use gauze strip or tape placed just caudal to upper canine teeth
  - pull nose toward cassette
  - tie gauze to table or around sandbag
- use gauze strip or tape placed just caudal to lower canine teeth
  - pull mandible to open mouth
  - tie gauze to table or around sandbag
- use gauze strips to rotate head
  - position the hard palate at a 45° angle to the table top
- the midline of the head should be parallel to the table top
- place pinnae of ears laterally
- endotracheal tube can be removed or remain in position
- pull tongue laterally away from the upper teeth

X-ray beam centering
- direct vertical beam on upper 3rd premolar tooth

Collimation
– include all teeth and paranasal sinuses

Comments
– positioning can be altered by further depressing the dog's nose
– angle X-ray beam caudorostrally if nose remains elevated
– can use roll of gauze or dental speculum to maintain open-mouth position
– breeds with short nose are difficult to position for this study
– can use pinnae as "handles" to assist in positioning head
– radiograph the opposite maxilla so a comparison study of the other upper dental arcade is available

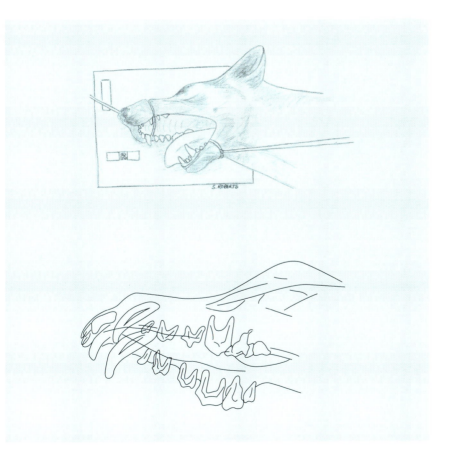

S. ROBERTS

Dental studies – oblique view of lower premolars and molars

Body
- place in sternal recumbency using a trough
- position body so sternum is laterally away from the lower arcade to be studied
- compression band across thorax or position sandbags lateral to the dog's body to maintain dorsoventral position

Forelimbs
- place limbs in a flexed position
- place sandbag across forelimbs

Hindlimbs
- place limbs in a neutral position

Head and neck
- place cassette on table top
- place head on cassette
- extend head in natural position
- rotate the dorsum of the head
- use gauze strip or tape placed just caudal to upper canine teeth
  - pull nose toward cassette
  - tie gauze to table or around sandbag
- use gauze strip or tape placed just caudal to lower canine teeth
  - pull mandible to open mouth
  - tie gauze to table or around sandbag
- use gauze strips to rotate head
  - position the hard palate at a 45° angle to the table top
- place pinnae of ears laterally
- endotracheal tube can be left in position
- pull tongue laterally away from the lower teeth

X-ray beam centering
- direct vertical beam into mouth centering on the 3rd lower premolar tooth

Collimation
– include all lower teeth

Comments
– radiograph the opposite half of the mandible so a comparison study is available
– breed type determines the length of the body of the mandible and the success in obtaining this view
– a shorter jaw is difficult to position parallel to the table top
– can use pinnae as "handles" to assist in positioning head
– can use roll of gauze or dental speculum to maintain open-mouth position

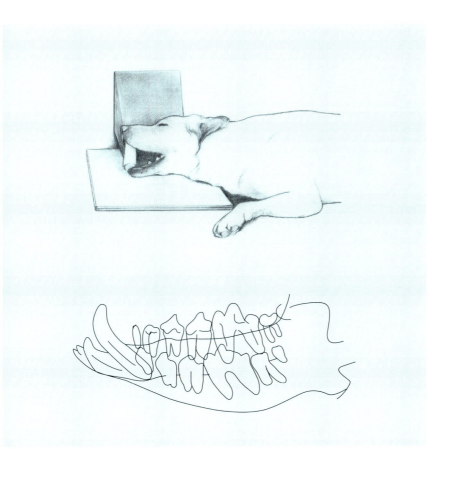

Dental studies – upper incisors

Body
- place in sternal recumbency using a trough
- position body so sternum is on midline
- compression band across thorax or position sandbags lateral to dog's body to maintain dorsoventral position

Forelimbs
- place limbs in an extended abducted position
- place sandbag across forelimbs

Hindlimbs
- place limbs in a neutral position

Head and neck
- place head on table top
- extend head in natural position
- open the mouth and place a corner of a non-sceen film into the mouth
- close mouth gently, since teeth striking the film may cause a pressure artifact or may even cut the paper film holder
- tongue and endotracheal tube are positioned beneath the film
- place pinnae of ears laterally

X-ray beam centering
- angle beam 20° to 30° rostrocaudally
- center on the dog's nose
- beam is directed perpendicular to the long axis of the incisors

Collimation
- include the incisor region

Comments

– it is possible to use a thin screened cassette for this study
– the film only need be inserted a short distance into the mouth
– maintain a 40" (100 cm) tube-film distance if using a screen system
– decrease tube-film distance to 30" (75 cm) if using a nonscreen system
– by angling the X-ray beam laterally, an oblique view can be obtained

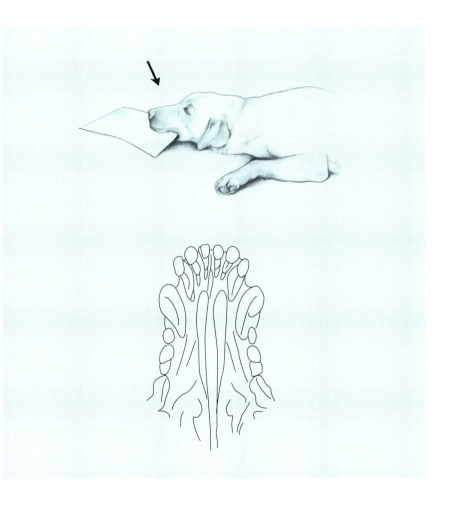

Dental studies – lower incisors

Body
- place in dorsal recumbency using a trough
- position body so sternum is on midline
- use a compression band across thorax or position sandbags latera
  to the dog's body to maintain ventrodorsal position

Forelimbs
- place limbs beside the thoracic wall
- place sandbag across forelimbs

Hindlimbs
- place limbs in a neutral position

Head and neck
- place head on table top
- extend head in natural position
- place one corner of non-screen film holder into mouth
- close mouth gently, since teeth striking the film may cause a
  pressure artifact or may even cut the paper film holder
- use gauze strip or tape placed over the rostral mandible to assist in
  positioning the mandible parallel to the table top
- place pinnae of ears laterally
- endotracheal tube can be left in position

X-ray beam centering
- angle beam 20° to 30° rostrocaudally
- center on the lower lip
- beam is directed perpendicular to the long axis of the incisors

Collimation
- include all lower incisors

Comments

- it is possible to use a thin screened cassette for this study
- the film only need be inserted a short distance into the mouth
- maintain a 40" (100 cm) tube-film distance if using a screen system
- decrease tube-film distance to 30" (75 cm) if using a non-sceen system
- by angling the X-ray beam laterally, an oblique view can be obtained (see drawing below)

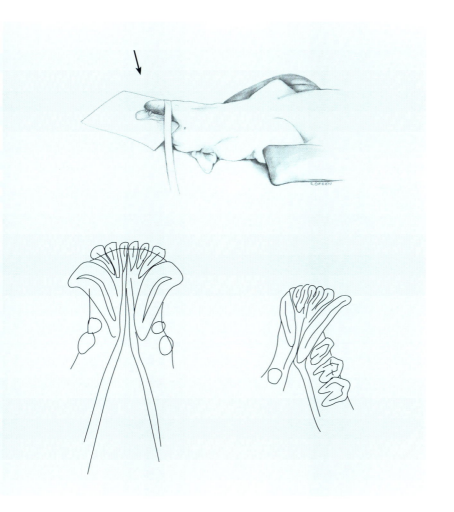

Pharyngeal Studies

Introduction
- air in the passages of the upper respiratory tract acts as a contrast agent and permits visualization of the soft structures of the pharyngeal area
- the study is usually limited to the lateral view since the cervical spine superimposes with the soft tissue structures on the ventrodorsal or dorsoventral view
- oblique views from the ventrodorsal may be helpful

Patient preparation
- consider removal of the endotracheal tube
- identify location of ears to insure they are not folded under the head

Anesthesia
- anesthesia is not required for most studies

Views
- recommended views
  - lateral with vertical beam
- special views
  - lateral with horizontal beam

X-ray Technique
– decrease kVp setting for soft tissues

Use of Grid
– a grid is not required for pharyngeal studies unless performed in a very large dog

Comments
– a rarely used study but often helpful in locating suspected mass lesions

Pharyngeal study – lateral view

Body
- position in
  - lateral recumbency
  - sternal recumbency
  - sitting or standing

Forelimbs
- position limbs caudally
- place sandbag across limbs or use tie-down ropes if recumbent

Hindlimbs
- place limbs in a neutral position

Head and neck
- with dog recumbent
  - place head and neck on cassette in an extended position
  - place sponge block under neck
  - place sponge block under nose
  - place sandbags against dorsum of neck
  - place pinnae of ears dorsally
- with dog in sternal recumbency
  - tape pinnae of ears dorsally
  - place head on large sponge block or hold nose up with a gloved hand
- with dog standing or sitting
  - extend head and neck

X-ray beam centering
- direct vertical or horizontal beam on center of neck

Collimation
- include all of pharyngeal region

Comments

– extend the head and neck to remove the ramus of the mandible from the pharyngeal region
– decrease the X-ray technique by 10 kVp because the study is of soft tissue
– may need to position the ears (pinnae) dorsally by taping

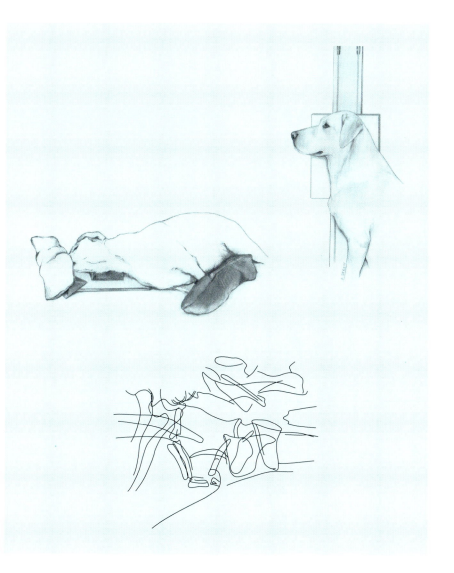

Notes

Spine

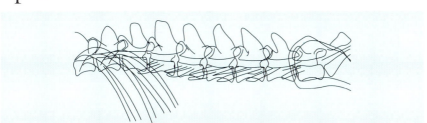

Spine

Introduction
- a most difficult group of studies to perform because of the character of the bones to be evaluated
- positioning of these "block-like", small bones with heavy bony processes, in addition to the radiolucent intervertebral discs, may be difficult
- clinical information such as breed and onset of clinical signs, as well as the severity and nature of neurologic deficits should suggest the region of the spine that should be more carefully evaluated on the radiograph
- it is a good protocol to radiograph the entire spine because it may be difficult accurately to localize the site of the lesion clinically

Patient preparation
- inspect haircoat for matted hair, debris, foreign bodies
- avoid unnecessary movement in positioning that might cause more injury to the spinal cord

Sedation or anesthesia
- not required for a survey study (patient with acute trauma)
- required for a definitive study

Studies
- regions of the spine are divided: occipito-atlanto-axial region, cervical spine, cervicothoracic spine, thoracic spine, thoracolumbar spine, lumbar spine, and lumbosacral spine

Views
- recommended views
  - ventrodorsal
  - lateral
- special views
  - stress views (dynamic radiography)
  - hyperextended (occipito-atlanto-axial region, and lumbo-sacral regions)
  - hyperflexed (caudal cervical, occipito-atlanto-axial region, and lumbosacral regions)
  - traction views (cervical region)
  - oblique views may permit better evaluation of the inter-vertebral foramina
  - special oblique view of the occipito-atlanto-axial region for odontoid process
  - open-mouth view for the odontoid process (p 68)

X-ray technique
- medium to low kVp may permit better evaluation

Use of grid
- required for patients measuring >11 cm

Special techniques
- use of compression paddle to shift soft tissue shadows away from the spine

Comments
- elevate cervical spine using sponges so it is parallel to the table top
- use sponges to elevate sternum and abdomen so that body is not rotated
- adequate evaluation of disk space width is limited to the central portion of the radiograph due to beam divergence peripherally on the radiograph

Spine – Occipito-atlanto-axial Region

Introduction
- injuries in this portion of the spine are often associated with congenital abnormalities, involving the odontoid process
- it is possible to cause additional injury to the spinal cord by excessive motion of the patient during radiography
- stress views are of value in patients with suspected instability but need to be performed carefully
- a different type of radiographic study is required in dogs suspected of having traumatic, neoplastic, or inflammatory disease

Patient preparation
- inspect haircoat for matted hair, debris, foreign bodies
- avoid unnecessary movement that might cause more injury to the spinal cord
- may be possible to radiograph patient strapped to a restraint board used to assist in transport and prevent further damage to the spinal cord

Sedation or anesthesia
- not required for a survey study
- required for a definitive study
- may be required to protect the dog from further injury

Views
- recommended views
  - ventrodorsal view
  - lateral view
- special views
- lateral stress views (dynamic radiography)
  - hyperextended
  - hyperflexed
  - basilar view for the occipital condyles (p 66, 112)
  - lateral view with rotation of head for the odontoid process (p 110)
  - open-mouth view for the odontoid process (p 68)

X-ray technique
- medium to low kVp may permit better evaluation

Use of grid
- usually not required for cervical spine except in a giant breed

Comments
- sponges required to elevate the spine so it is parallel to the table top
- use sponges to elevate sternum and abdomen so that body is not rotated

Occipito-atlanto-axial region – lateral view

Body
- place in lateral recumbency
- place a sponge beneath the sternum to avoid rotation of the body
- place compression band across thorax or abdomen

Forelimbs
- extend limbs caudally
- place sponge block between limbs
- place sandbag across forelimbs

Hindlimbs
- place limbs in a neutral position

Head and neck
- place cassette on table top
- place head on cassette
- extend head cranially in neutral position
- place sponge under neck
- place sponge wedge under nose so head is parallel to the table top
- insure that a line marking the midsagittal place is parallel to the table top
- insure that a line drawn between the medial canthi of the eyes is perpendicular to the table top
- place sandbag against top of head
- place pinnae of ears dorsally
- endotracheal tube can remain in position

X-ray beam centering
- direct vertical beam on base of skull

Collimation
- include base of skull and first cervical segments

Comments
- positioning can be altered by hyperextending or hyperflexing the head
- position sandbags dorsal and ventral to the head to assist in stress studies
- can use pinnae as "handles" to assist in positioning head

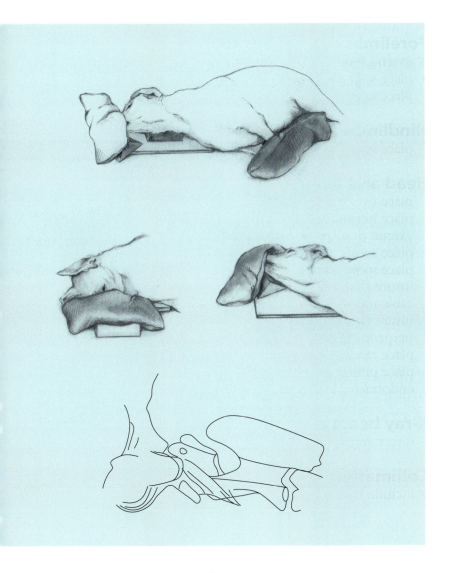

Occipito-atlanto-axial region – ventrodorsal view

Body
- place on pad or in trough in dorsal recumbency
- use compression band across thorax or abdomen
- palpate sternum (xyphoid process) on midline to insure correct position

Forelimbs
- place limbs beside the thoracic wall
- place sandbag across forelimbs or use tie-down ropes

Hindlimbs
- place limbs in a frog-leg flexed position

Head and neck
- place cassette on table top
- place head and neck on cassette
- place head so that the nose is pointed upwards, with sandbags positioned laterally and rostrally
- locate pinnae of ears laterally
- endotracheal tube may need to be removed

X-ray beam centering
- direct vertical beam on C1

Collimation
- include base of skull and first cervical segments

Comments

- positioning can be altered by hyperextending or hyperflexing the head
- position sandbags dorsal and ventral to the head to assist in stress studies
- can use pinnae as "handles" to assist in positioning head
- stress studies can be made by positioning the head to the right or left (see drawings below)

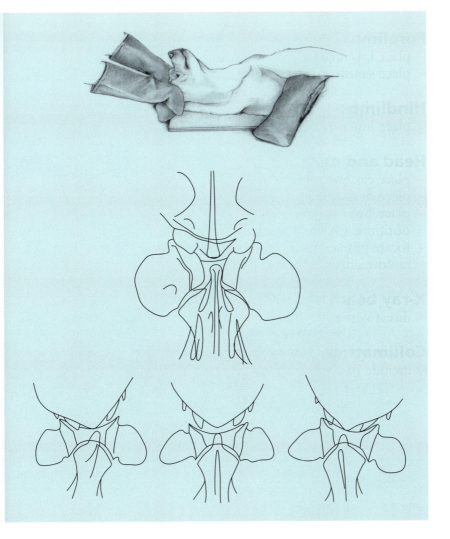

Occipito-atlanto-axial region – lateral view for odontoid process

Body
- place in lateral recumbency
- place a sponge beneath the sternum to avoid rotation of the body
- place compression band across thorax or abdomen

Forelimbs
- position limbs caudally
- place sponge block between limbs
- place sandbag across forelimbs

Hindlimbs
- place limbs in a neutral position

Head and neck
- place cassette on table top
- place neck on cassette
- extend head cranially
- place sponge under neck
- rotate head toward a dorsoventral position
- place sandbag against top of head
- place pinnae of ears dorsally
- endotracheal tube can remain in position

X-ray beam centering
- direct vertical beam on base of skull

Collimation
- include base of skull and first cervical segments

Comments

– can use pinnae as "handles" to assist in positioning head
– a rotational view allows good evaluation of the odontoid process
– comparison of the oblique views allows for evaluation of the occipital condyles

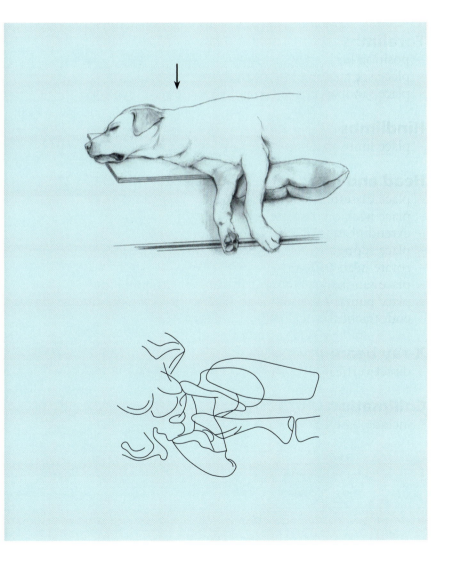

Occipito-atlanto-axial region – fronto-occipital view

Body
- place in dorsal recumbency using a trough
- position sternum on midline
- place compression band across thorax or abdomen, or position sandbags lateral to dog's body to maintain ventrodorsal position

Forelimbs
- place limbs along side of thorax
- place sandbag across forelimbs or use tie-down rope

Hindlimbs
- place limbs in a neutral frog-leg position

Head and neck
- place cassette on table top
- position head on cassette
- position head with nose pointing upwards
- wrap gauze strip or tape around dorsum of nose
  - pull nose caudally
  - angle hard palate caudally 30°– 45° to table top
  - tie gauze strip or tape to table edge or wrap around sandbags
- place sandbags against both sides of head
- place sandbag against top of head
- place pinnae of ears laterally
- endotracheal tube can be removed or remain in position

X-ray beam centering
- direct vertical beam between eyes

Collimation
- include base of skull

Comments
- can use pinnae as "handles" to assist in positioning head in awake patient
- decrease X-ray technique appropriately
- the shape of the head may influence positioning for this view

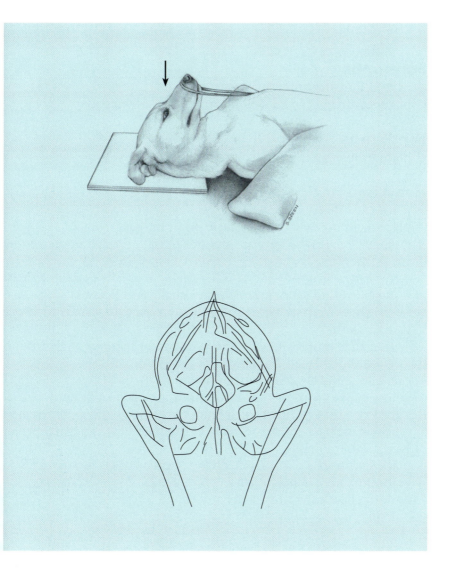

Occipito-atlanto-axial region – open-mouth view for odontoid process

Body
- place in dorsal recumbency using a trough
- position sternum on midline
- place compression band across thorax or abdomen or position sandbags lateral to dog's body to maintain ventrodorsal position

Forelimbs
- extend limbs in a neutral position
- place sandbag across forelimbs or use tie-down rope

Hindlimbs
- place limbs in a neutral frog-leg position

Head and neck
- place cassette on table top
- place head on cassette with nose pointing upwards
- wrap gauze strip or tape around nose just caudal to upper canine teeth
    - tie gauze strip or tape to side of table cranially and laterally or wrap around sandbags placed cranially and laterally
- wrap gauze strip or tape around lower jaw just caudal to lower canine teeth
    - tie gauze strip or tape caudally to end of table or wrap around a sandbag placed caudally
- pull gauze tightly until mouth opens
- adjust gauze strips or tape until mouth is open as desired
- adjust position of head so the line that bisects the angle created by the hard palate and the body of the mandible is perpendicular to the table top
- place sandbags against both sides of head
- place pinnae of ears laterally
- endotracheal tube must be removed

X-ray beam centering
– direct vertical beam to bisect angle between the hard palate and the lower jaw

Collimation
–   include tympanic bullae, C1, and odontoid process of C2

Comments
– positioning of head is breed-dependent
– position the head carefully in patients suspected of trauma
– decrease the X-ray technique appropriately

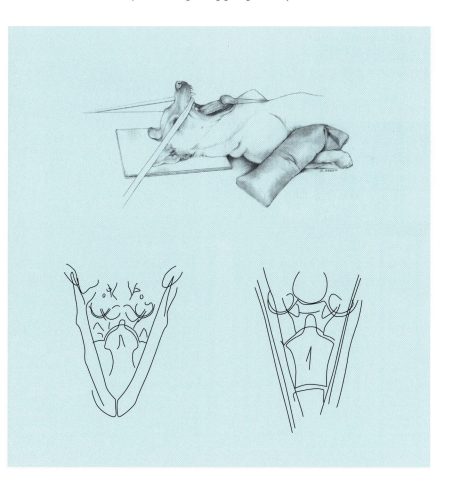

Spine – Cervical Region

Introduction
- these patients are usually suspected of having either acute or chronic disc disease and the positioning is particularly important to permit close evaluation of the character of each disc space
- character of the end plates and visualization of the spinal canal through the intervertebral foramina just dorsal to the disc spaces is also important
- other less definitive studies are required in dogs suspected of traumatic, neoplastic, or inflammatory disease
- stress views are valuable in evaluation of patients with suspected cervical instability

Patient preparation
- inspect haircoat for matted hair, debris, foreign bodies
- avoid unnecessary movement of the cervical spine which might cause more injury to the spinal cord

Sedation or anesthesia
- not required for a survey study
- required for a definitive study

Views
- recommended views
  - neutral ventrodorsal view
  - lateral view
- special views
  - lateral stress views (dynamic radiography)
    - hyperextended
    - hyperflexed
  - traction
  - oblique views from the ventrodorsal position

X-ray technique
– medium to low kVp may permit better evaluation of bone

Use of grid
– usually not required for cervical spine except in a large or giant breed

Comments
– sponges required to make the spine parallel to table top
– use sponges to elevate sternum and abdomen so that body is not rotated

Cervical spine – lateral view

Body
- place in lateral recumbency
- place compression band across thorax or abdomen

Forelimbs
- extend limbs caudally
- place sandbag across forelimbs or use tie-down rope

Hindlimbs
- place limbs in a neutral position

Head and neck
- place cassette on table top
- place head and neck on cassette
- extend head cranially
- place sponge block under neck
- place sponge wedge under nose
- place pinnae of ears dorsally
- place sandbag over nose

X-ray beam centering
- direct vertical beam on center of neck (note that the cervical spine is more ventral than suspected)

Collimation
- include all of cervical spine

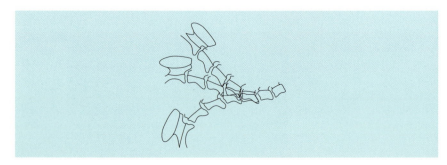

Comments

– stress views can be made with the head positioned into a hyper-extended or hyperflexed view (see drawings below)
– traction views can be made with the spine in neutral position by pulling on the head with gloved hands
– because of the increase in tissue thickness make a separate radiograph of C7-T1 by increasing the X-ray technique by 10 kVp
– can use pinnae as "handles" to assist in positioning head

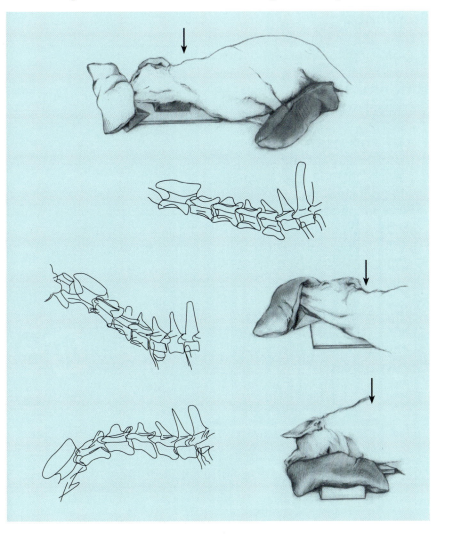

Cervical spine – ventrodorsal view

Body
- place on pad or in trough in dorsal recumbency
- place compression band across thorax or abdomen
- palpate sternum (xyphoid process) on midline to insure correct position

Forelimbs
- place limbs beside the thoracic wall
- place sandbag across forelimbs or use tie-down rope

Hindlimbs
- place in frog-leg position

Head and neck
- place cassette on table top
- place head and neck on casette
- extend head in natural position
- place sponge beneath the neck to elevate the spine so it is parallel to the table top
- place head so the nose is pointed upwards, with sandbags positioned laterally and rostrally
- it may be helpful to elevate the head on a block

X-ray beam centering
- direct vertical beam on center of cervical region

Collimation
- include base of skull and entire cervical spine

Comments
– remove endotracheal tube just prior to exposure
– if nose is improperly positioned next to the table top, the base of the skull will overlie the first cervical segments and prevent their evaluation
– with the head and neck elevated a vertical beam can be used
– if the head rests on the table top, the beam should be angled 15° caudorostrally

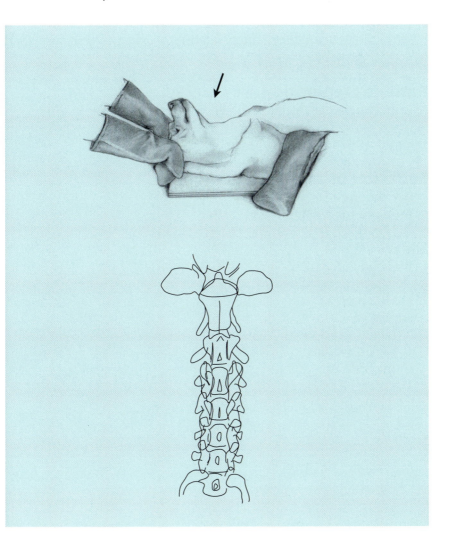

Spine – Cervicothoracic region

Introduction
- these patients are usually suspected of having either acute or chronic disc disease or developmental lesions associated with a cervical spondylopathy
- character of the end plates and visualization of the spinal canal through the intervertebral foramina just dorsal to the disc spaces is difficult because of the overlying shoulders
- stress views are valuable in evaluation of patients with suspected cervical instability

Patient preparation
- inspect haircoat for matted hair, debris, foreign bodies
- avoid unnecessary movement of the cervical spine which might cause more injury to the spinal cord

Sedation or anesthesia
- not required for a survey study
- required for a definitive study

Views
- recommended views
  - ventrodorsal view with angled beam
  - lateral view
- special views
  - lateral stress views (dynamic radiography)
  - hyperextended
  - hyperflexed

X-ray technique
– high kVp is required for penetration

Use of grid
– usually not required for cervical spine except in a large or giant breed

Comments
– sponges required to make the spine parallel to the table top
– use sponges to elevate sternum and abdomen so that body is not rotated

Cervicothoracic spine – lateral view

Body
- place in lateral recumbency
- place compression band across thorax or abdomen

Forelimbs
- extend limbs caudally
- place sandbag across forelimbs or use tie-down rope

Hindlimbs
- place limbs in a neutral extended position

Head and neck
- place cassette on table top
- place neck on cassette
- extend head cranially
- place sponge block under neck
- place sponge wedge under nose
- place pinnae of ears dorsally

X-ray beam centering
- direct vertical beam on shoulders
- the cervicothoracic junction is located ventrally in the neck

Collimation
- include C6–7 and T1–2

Comments
- stress views can be made with the head positioned into a hyperextension or hyperflexion
- because of the increase in tissue thickness increase the X-ray technique by 10 kVp
- can use pinnae as "handles" to assist in positioning head

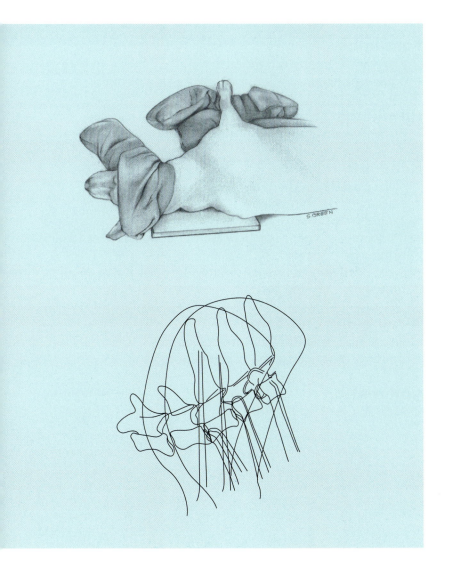

Cervicothoracic spine – ventrodorsal view

Body
- place in dorsal recumbency on pad or in trough
- place a compression band across thorax
- palpate sternum (xyphoid process) on midline to insure correct position

Forelimbs
- place limbs beside the thoracic wall
- place sandbag across limbs or use tie-down ropes

Hindlimbs
- place in neutral frog-leg position

Head and neck
- place cassette on the table
- place neck on the cassette
- extend head in natural position
- if possible, place sponge beneath the head and neck to elevate the spine so it is parallel to the table top
- place head so the nose is pointed upwards, with sandbags positioned laterally and rostrally

X-ray beam centering
- direct beam at a 20° caudorostral angle
- center on the cervicothoracic junction

Collimation
- include C6–7 and T1–2

Comments
– partially retract the endotracheal tube just prior to exposure
– with the head elevated a more nearly vertical beam can be used

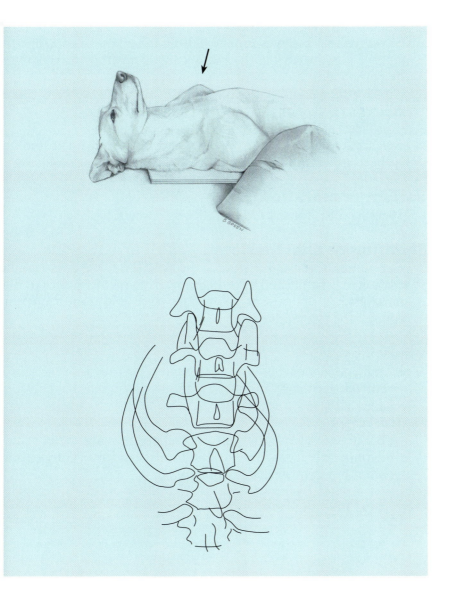

Spine – Thoracic Region

Introduction
- include in a complete spinal survey
- it is possible to make only an abbreviated study of a particular region of interest ("cone down")
- the ventrodorsal view is usually of little value but it is possible to improve it by increasing the kVp setting in an effort to penetrate the dense mediastinal tissues on this view
- character of the end plates and width of the disc space is more difficult to evaluate than in other parts of the spine
- stress views are not possible in the thoracic region
- often follows a thoracic study in which an unexplained finding has been noted in the spine

Patient preparation
- inspect haircoat for matted hair, debris, foreign bodies

Sedation or anesthesia
- not required for a survey study
- sedation may be needed to protect dog from further injury to the spinal cord
- required for a definitive study

Views
- recommended views
  - ventrodorsal view
  - lateral view
- special views
  - oblique views from the ventrodorsal position may be of value
  - uncommonly it may be of value to make a dorsoventral study with the dog in sternal recumbency

X-ray technique
– higher kVp is necessary to penetrate the mediastinal structures

Use of grid
– required in medium, large, and giant breeds

Comments
– it is difficult to position the thoracic spine parallel to the table top for a VD or DV study because the thoracic spine is not parallel to the long axis of the body but is more ventral in the cranial portion of the thorax and more dorsal in the caudal portion of the thorax
– may be helpful to angle the central beam

Thoracic spine – lateral view

Body
- place cassette in position
- place body in lateral recumbency
- place a sponge wedge beneath the sternum
- use a compression band across thorax or abdomen

Forelimbs
- extend limbs cranially
- place a sponge block between the elbows
- place sandbag across forelimbs or use tie-down rope

Hindlimbs
- place limbs in a neutral or extended position
- place a sponge block between the stifle joints
- place sandbag across hindlimbs or use tie-down rope

Head and neck
- place head in neutral position
- place sponge block beneath the neck
- place sandbag over neck

X-ray beam centering
- direct vertical beam on the dorsal thorax

Collimation
- include all of thoracic spine

Comments
- a view centered on the thoracolumbar region is often made because of frequent disc lesions at this site
- may make the study with patient lying on either right or left side
- no value in making both lateral views
- important to include thoracic spinous processes in patients in which multiple myeloma or trauma is suspected

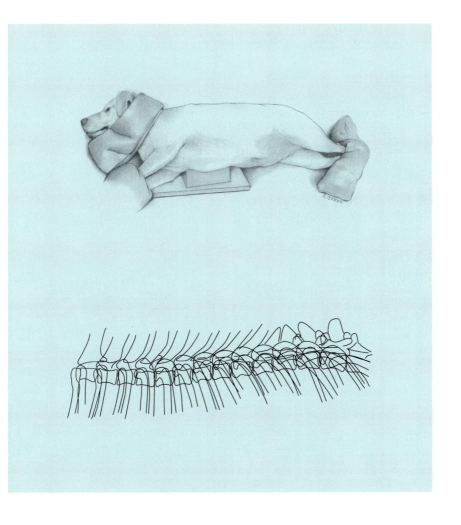

Thoracic spine – ventrodorsal view

Body
- place cassette in position
- place body in dorsal recumbency on pad or in trough
- use a compression band across abdomen
- palpate sternum (xyphoid process) on midline to insure correct position

Forelimbs
- extend limbs cranially
- place sandbag across forelimbs or use tie-down rope

Hindlimbs
- place in frog-leg position
- place sandbags across hindlimbs or use tie-down rope

Head and neck
- extend head in natural position

X-ray beam centering
- direct vertical beam on center of thoracic region just cranial to xyphoid

Collimation
- include entire thoracic spine

Comments

- may see disc spaces on the ventrodorsal view more clearly using a slightly angled caudocranial beam
- it is more difficult to achieve a good ventrodorsal position in dogs with a deep chest because of the narrowness and increased depth of the thorax
- a dorsal mass lesion may make positioning in dorsal recumbency difficult and necessitating dorsoventral positioning
- it is possible to make a dorsoventral view of the thoracic spine using the position describing that view for the thorax (p 26)
- a dorsoventral study for the thoracic spine is usually not considered as diagnostic because of the increase in the object-film distance

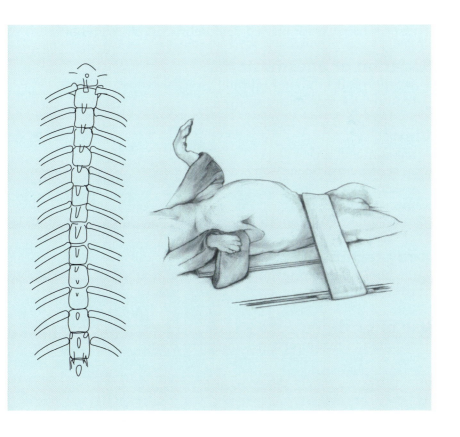

Spine – Thoracolumbar Region

Introduction
- this is a highly recommended additional study in dogs with spinal disease because of the high frequency of disc herniation involving these discs
- it should be an additional view to a routine study of the thoracic and/or lumbar spine
- the ventrodorsal view is often of little value because of overlying soft tissue shadows and difficult positioning
- correct body positioning is important, making the use of sponge wedges and blocks imperative
- stress views are not used

Patient preparation
- inspect haircoat for matted hair, debris, and foreign bodies

Sedation or anesthesia
- sedation is helpful in positioning for a survey study
- required for a definitive study

Views
- recommended views
    - ventrodorsal view
    - lateral view
- special views
    - oblique views from the ventrodorsal position may be of value

X-ray technique
- medium kVp settings may make identification of calcified disc tissue easier

Use of grid
- required in medium, large, and giant breeds

Comments
- overlying rib shadows compromise visualization of disc spaces on the lateral view
- in making the lateral view, it is possible to make several exposures on the same film varying the positioning of the dog slightly
- in making the ventrodorsal view, it is possible to reposition the X-ray tube to achieve slight angulation keeping the beam within the plane of the midline of the dog
- may be helpful to angle the central beam

Thoracolumbar spine – lateral view

Body
- place cassette in position
- place body in lateral recumbency
- place a sponge wedge beneath the sternum

Forelimbs
- extend limbs cranially
- place a sponge block between the elbows
- place sandbag across forelimbs or use tie-down rope

Hindlimbs
- extend limbs caudally
- place a sponge block between the stifle joints
- place sandbags across hind limbs or use tie-down rope

Head and neck
- place head in neutral position
- place sandbag over neck

X-ray beam centering
- direct vertical beam where the last rib joins the spine

Collimation
- collimate closely so more than one exposure can be made on a film

Comments

- the study may be made with the patient lying on either the right or left side
- there may be value in making both lateral views because it requires repositioning of the patient and may shift soft tissue shadows
- most common error is positioning without elevating the sternum

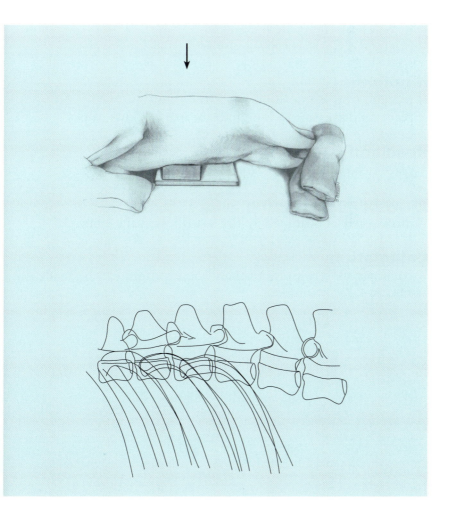

Thoracolumbar spine – ventrodorsal view

Body
- place cassette in position
- place body in dorsal recumbency on pad or in trough
- place compression band across the caudal abdomen
- palpate sternum (xyphoid process) on midline to insure correct position

Forelimbs
- extend limbs cranially
- place sandbag across forelimbs or use tie-down ropes

Hindlimbs
- place in frog-leg position
- place sandbags across hindlimbs or use tie-down ropes

Head and neck
- place head in neutral position

X-ray beam centering
- direct vertical beam where the last rib joins the spine

Collimation
- collimate closely so more than one exposure can be made on a film

Comments
- insure that positioning devices are shifted so as not to be within the primary beam
- most common error is not correcting patient obliquity
- may see disc spaces on this view more clearly using a slightly angled caudocranial beam
- it is more difficult to make this view if the dog has a deep chest
- it is possible to make this view with the dog in sternal recumbency (p 26)

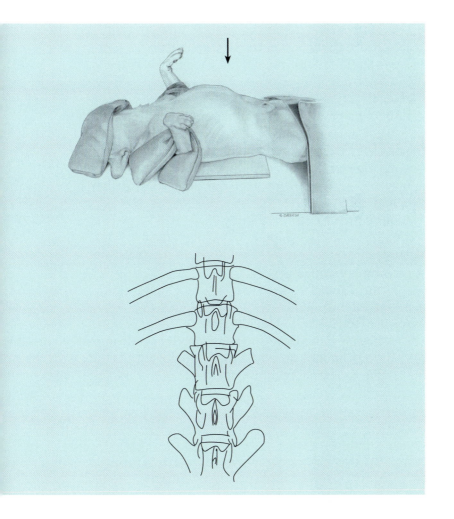

Spine – Lumbar Region

Introduction
– this is a most common study following trauma or in search for possible inflammatory or neoplastic disease
– other examinations are in search of suspected disc disease and the radiographic projection of each disc space is important
– determination of the character of the end plates and width of the disc space is more easily ascertained in the lumbar region than in other regions of the spine because of the absence of the ribs
– the lumbosacral region is unique anatomically and the radiographic examination is treated separately
– stress views are not possible in the lumbar region

Patient preparation
– inspect haircoat for matted hair, debris, foreign bodies

Sedation or anesthesia
– not required for a survey study
– may be required to protect the dog from further injury to the spinal cord
– required for a definitive study

Views
– recommended views
  – ventrodorsal
  – lateral
– special views
  – oblique views from the ventrodorsal position may be of value
  – it may be indicated to make a dorsoventral study with the dog in sternal recumbency

X-ray technique
– use routine kVp

Use of grid
– required in medium, large, and giant breeds

Comments
– lateral view often lacks diagnostic quality because the dog is oblique or the beam is centered on the abdomen instead of the lumbar spine

Lumbar spine – lateral view

Body
- place cassette in position
- place body in lateral recumbency
- place a sponge wedge beneath the sternum
- place compression band across thorax

Forelimbs
- extend limbs cranially
- place a sponge block between the elbows
- place sandbag across forelimbs or use tie-down rope

Hindlimbs
- extend limbs candally
- position the dependent limb slightly cranial to the upper limb
- place a sponge block between the stifle joints
- place sandbag across hindlimbs or use tie-down rope

Head and neck
- place head in neutral position
- place sandbag over neck

X-ray beam centering
- direct vertical beam on lumbar spine

Collimation
- include all of lumbar spine

Comments
– may make the study with either the right or left side next to the table top
– little value in making both lateral views

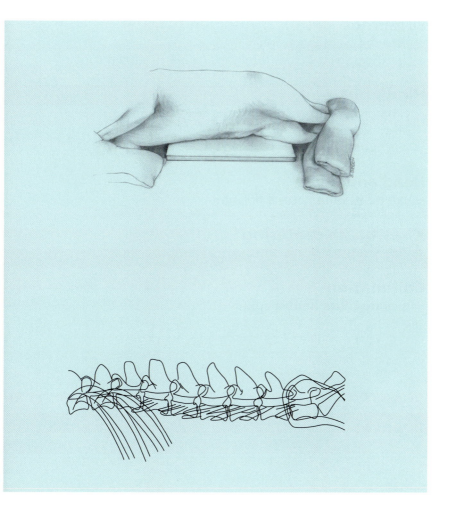

Lumbar spine – ventrodorsal view

Body
- place cassette in position
- place body in dorsal recumbency on pad or in trough
- place compression band across thorax
- palpate sternum (xyphoid process) on midline to insure correct position
- palpate pelvis to insure its position

Forelimbs
- place limbs in extension
- place sandbags across forelimbs or use tie-down rope

Hindlimbs
- extend caudally or leave in frog-leg position
- place sandbags across hindlimbs or use tie-down rope or hold with gloved hands

Head and neck
- extend head in natural position

X-ray beam centering
- direct vertical beam on center of lumbar region

Collimation
- include entire lumbar spine

Comments
- a dog may have a dorsal lesion making dorsal recumbency difficult
- it is possible to make a dorsoventral view with the dog in sternal recumbency, but there is an increase in the object-film distance (p 46)
- the ventrodorsal view is not satisfactory to evaluate the lumbosacral junction
- use frog-leg positioning of the hindlimbs in trauma cases with suspect femoral or pelvic fractures

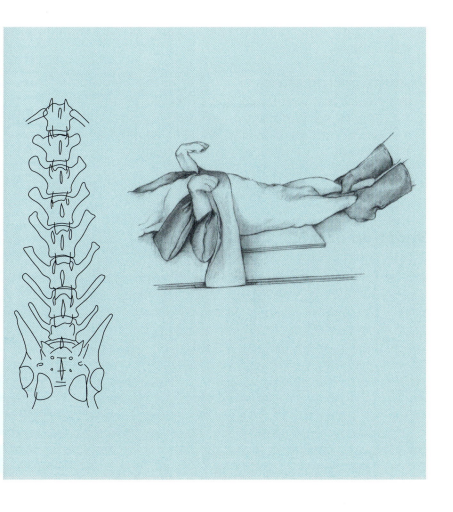

Spine – Lumbosacral Region

Introduction
- this is a common study often made in addition to the study of the lumbar spine or pelvis
- specific congenital, developmental, inflammatory, degenerative, and neoplastic lesions center on the lumbosacral junction, especially involving that disc
- the ventrodorsal view is of greater value if the beam is angled
- determination of the character of the end plates and width of the lumbosacral disc space is particularly important
- stress views are an important portion of the study in the evaluation of stability

Patient preparation
- inspect haircoat for matted hair, debris, foreign bodies
- a fecal-filled rectum compromises study quality
- a distended urinary bladder is actually helpful since it provides a background of uniform soft tissue density on the ventrodorsal view
- note the position of the tail is outside of the radiation field in all views

Sedation or anesthesia
- not required for a survey study
- required for a definitine study including stress views

Views
- recommended views
  - ventrodorsal with a caudocranially angled beam
  - lateral
- special views
  - lateral stress views with the hindlimbs
    - hyperextended
    - hyperflexed
  - a dorsoventral view can be made with the dog in sternal recumbency with the hindlimbs in a hyperflexed position

X-ray technique
- an increase of 10 kVp is necessary because of the increased amount of bone tissue

Use of grid
- required in medium, large, and giant breeds

Comments
- lead sheets obtained from a discarded apron are useful to shield the testicles of a male dog from radiation

Lumbosacral spine – lateral view

Body
- place in lateral recumbency
- place a sponge wedge beneath the sternum
- place compression band across thorax

Forelimbs
- extend limbs cranially
- place sandbags across forelimbs or use tie-down rope

Hindlimbs
- 3 positions of the limbs are utilized
    - neutral
    - hyperflexed
    - hyperextended
- place cassette in position
- place sponge between the stifle joints
- place sandbags across hindlimbs or use tie-down rope
- place sandbag adjacent to dog's back
- place sandbag over tail

Head and neck
- place head in neutral position
- place sandbag over neck

X-ray beam centering
- direct vertical beam on lumbosacral junction

Collimation
- include last lumbar segments and part of the pelvis

Comments

– study made with the hindlimbs in 3 positions (see drawings below)
  – neutral with hindlimbs positioned 90° to the spinal column
  – hyperflexed, with sandbags holding hindlimbs flexed as far cranially as possible
  – hyperextended, with sandbags holding hindlimbs extended as far caudally as possible
– may make the study with the patient lying on either the right or left side
– no value in making both lateral views

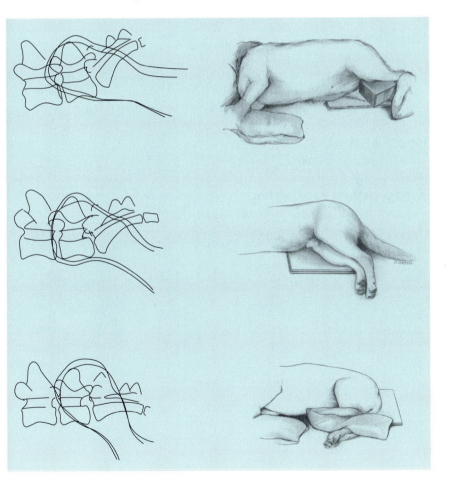

Lumbosacral spine – ventrodorsal view

Body
- place in dorsal recumbency on pad or in trough
- place compression band across thorax
- palpate sternum (xyphoid process) on midline to insure correct position of the body

Forelimbs
- place in neutral position
- place sandbags across forelimbs or use tie-down rope

Hindlimbs
- place cassette in position
- place limbs caudally in a partially flexed position (frog-leg) or fully extended
- place sandbags across hindlimbs or use tie-down rope

Head and neck
- extend head in natural position

X-ray beam centering
- direct beam angled 30° caudocranially
- center on lumbosacral junction

Collimation
- include caudal lumbar segments and part of the pelvis

Comments
- observe that tail is outside the radiation field
- it is possible to make a dorsoventral view with the dog in sternal recumbency using a craniocaudally angled beam

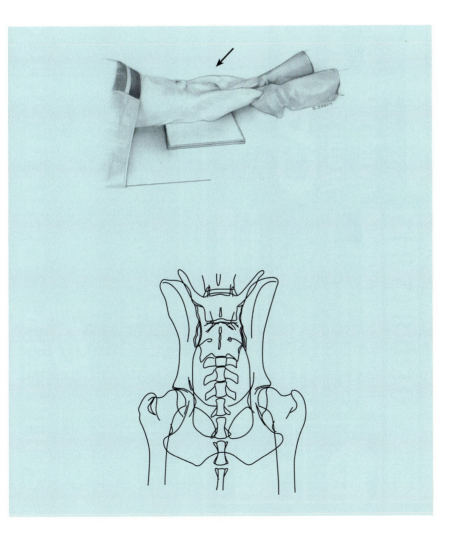

Notes

Pelvic Region

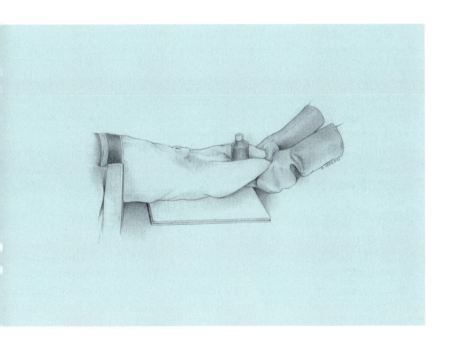

Pelvic Region

Introduction
- most studies of the pelvis and hip joints are performed to evaluate acutely detected pain or lameness
- detection of the type of fracture/luxation following injury is critical in determining the type of treatment required
- a special type of fracture seen in the immature patient is the slipped capital epiphysis
- other less common reasons for examination include congenital, inflammatory, neoplastic, and degenerative lesions
- a large and important group of patients studied are those under evaluation for the presence of hip dysplasia
- while most trauma patients are evaluated awake, hip dysplasia studies are better made as a prescheduled study in a sedated or anesthetized patient in an effort to achieve the best positioning

Patient preparation
- inspect haircoat for matted hair, debris, or foreign bodies
- rectal contents greatly compromise evaluation of the sacroiliac joints, sacrum, and the pubic bones on the ventrodorsal view
- testicles may be covered with lead shield in non-trauma patients
- control the position of the tail so it remains outside the primary radiation field

Sedation or anesthesia
- not required for a post-trauma study unless patient is in excessive pain
- highly recommended when evaluating the hip joints for the presence of dysplasia or other prescheduled patients

Views for routine studies
- recommended views
  - ventrodorsal
  - lateral
- special views
  - lateral view of the hip joint made with the pelvis oblique and the femur parallel to the table top

Views for hip dysplasia studies
- recommended views
  - ventrodorsal with limbs extended
- special views
  - ventrodorsal with limbs flexed ("frog-leg") view
  - ventrodorsal with limbs extended using a fulcrum technique
  - ventrodorsal with limbs perpendicular to table top using a distraction technique

X-ray technique
- routine settings are adequate

Use of grid
- required in medium, large, and giant breeds in both ventrodorsal and lateral views of the pelvis
- usually not required in lateral view of the hip joint

Comments
- trauma patients are difficult to position because of pain and / or nature of injury
- strive for similiar positioning of both hindlimbs so that projections of the two limbs are similar; avoid achieving an extended position for one limb and a flexed position for the other limb

Pelvis and hip joints – lateral view

Body
- place in lateral recumbency
- place a sponge wedge beneath the sternum
- place compression band across thorax

Forelimbs
- extend limbs cranially
- place sandbag across forelimbs

Head and neck
- place head in neutral position
- place sandbag over neck

Hindlimbs
- place cassette in position
- place limbs in a neutral position
- position the dependent limb cranial to the upper limb
- place a sponge block between the stifle joints
- place sandbag across hindlimbs or use tie-down rope

X-ray beam centering
- direct vertical beam on hip joints

Collimation
- include pelvis, hip joints, and proximal femurs

Comments

- study can be made with the patient lying on either the right or left side
- little value in making both lateral views
- strive for a very slightly oblique projection of the pelvis so that hip joints are not superimposed
- a particularly valuable study in the determination of the relationship of the femoral head to the acetabulum can be made with the pelvis in perfect lateral position and the beam directed 20° in a caudocranial direction, producing a radiograph in which the hip joints and femora are not superimposed (see drawings)
- the greatest value of this view is to determining the presence of a luxated hip or fractured pelvis and to evaluate the caudal lumbar and lumbosacral spine

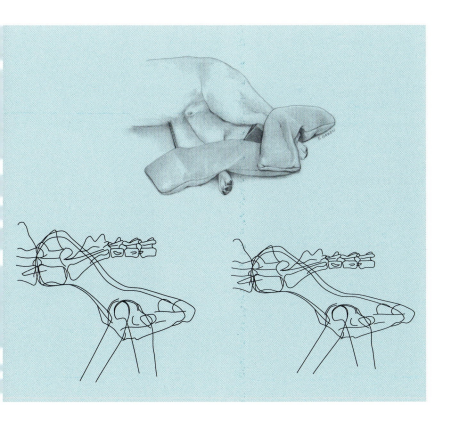

Pelvis and hip joints – ventrodorsal view

Body
- place in dorsal recumbency on pad or in trough
- use a compression band across thorax
- palpate sternum (xyphoid process) on midline to insure correct position

Forelimbs
- extend limbs cranially
- place sandbags across forelimbs

Head and neck
- extend head in natural position

Hindlimbs
- place cassette in position
- extend limbs caudally or place in frog-leg position
- place sandbags across hindlimbs or use tie-down rope
- most important to have hindlimbs in similar position

X-ray beam centering
- direct vertical beam on pelvis

Collimation
- include pelvis, both hip joints, and proximal femurs

Comments

- a dorsal lesion makes dorsal recumbency difficult, and dorso-ventral positioning with the dog in sternal recumbency may be necessary
- the limbs may be in either an extended or flexed position (p 46)
- this view is not satisfactory for evaluation of the lumbosacral junction
- comparison views can be made with the hindlimbs extended and with the hindlimbs flexed, to permit evaluation of lesions in the proximal femur or acetabula
- remove tail from radiation field

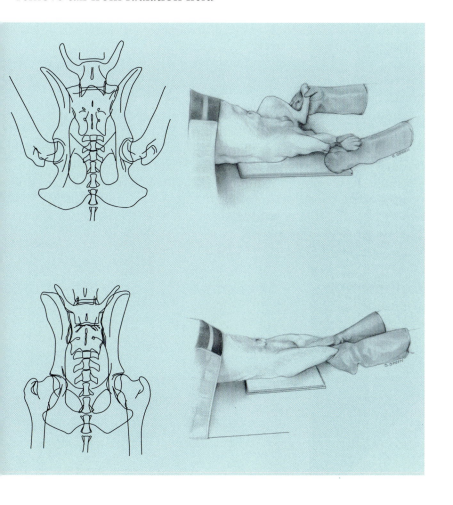

Hip joints – lateral view

Body
– place on pad in lateral recumbency with affected hip on table top
– use a compression band across thorax

Forelimbs
– extend limbs cranially
– place sandbags across forelimbs or use tie-down rope

Head and neck
– extend head in natural position
– place sandbag over neck

Hindlimbs
– place cassette in position
– abduct uppermost limb until femur is perpendicular to the table top, removing it from the radiation field
– secure uppermost limb by tie-down rope to tube stand or table edge or to sandbag or use a gloved hand
– extend lower hindlimb and place sandbag across or use tie-down rope or gloved hand

X-ray beam centering
– direct vertical beam on hip joint

Collimation
– include hip joint

Comments
- it may be necessary to angle the beam 10° to 20 ° distoproximally if the upper limb cannot be abducted sufficiently to remove it from the radiation field
- hold tail outside radiation field with sandbag

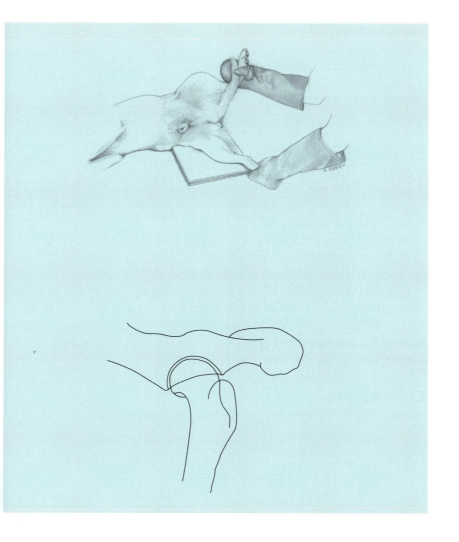

Hip dysplasia study – ventrodorsal view with limbs extended

Body
- place in dorsal recumbency on pad or in trough
- use a compression band across thorax
- palpate sternum (xyphoid process) on midline to insure correct position

Forelimbs
- extend limbs cranially
- place sandbags across forelimbs

Head and neck
- extend head in natural position

Hindlimbs
- place cassette in position
- extend limbs caudally
- place sandbags across hindlimbs or use tie-down rope or hold feet with gloved hands
- position both hindlimbs in a similar manner
- position so hindlimbs are extended so they are parallel to a line representing a continuation of the spine
- position the hindlimbs in internal rotation with patellas as near midline of each limb as is possible

X-ray beam centering
- direct vertical beam on pelvis

Collimation
- include pelvis, both hip joints, femurs, and stifle joints

Comments
– avoid having limbs abducted or in external rotation
– remove tail from radiation field
– use a cassette size that permits inclusion of the stifle joints

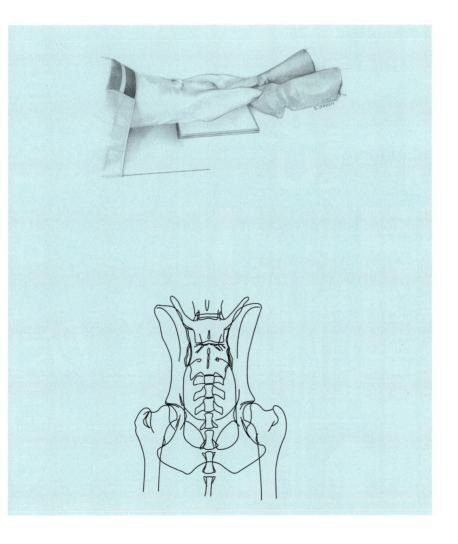

Hip dysplasia study – ventrodorsal view with limbs flexed ("frog-leg")

Body
– place in dorsal recumbency on pad or in trough
– use a compression band across thorax
– palpate sternum (xyphoid process) on midline to insure correct position

Forelimbs
– extend limbs cranially
– place sandbags across forelimbs

Head and neck
– extend head in natural position

Hindlimbs
– place cassette in position
– place limbs in maximum flexion in frog-leg position
– place sandbags across hindlimbs
– position hindlimbs in a similar manner

X-ray beam centering
– direct vertical beam on pelvis

Collimation
– include pelvis, both hip joints, and proximal femurs

Comments

- flexed position places the stifle joints cranial and lateral to the hip joints
- this is a more comfortable position for a dog with painful secondary joint disease of the hip joints
- remove tail from radiation field using sandbags

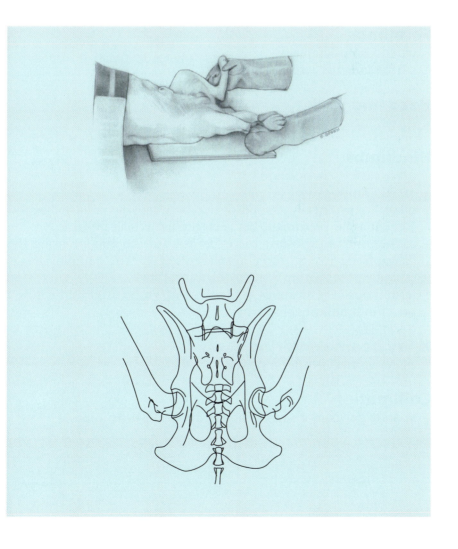

Hip dysplasia study – ventrodorsal view using fulcrum technique

Body
– place in dorsal recumbency on pad or in trough
– use a compression band across thorax
– palpate sternum (xyphoid process) on midline to insure correct position

Forelimbs
– extend limbs cranially
– place sandbags across forelimbs

Head and neck
– extend head in natural position

Hindlimbs
– place cassette in position
– extend limbs caudally
– place a cylindrically shaped device between the stifle joints and force it as far proximally between the limbs as is possible
– at the time of exposure, force feet toward the midline using the fulcrum device to force displacement of the femoral heads laterally potentiating a stage of subluxation
– hold limbs in position by using tie-down rope or gloved hands
– position hindlimbs similarly

X-ray beam centering
– direct vertical beam on pelvis

Collimation
– include pelvis, both hip joints, femurs, and stifle joints

Comments
- size of fulcrum device should approximate the diameter of the upper hindlimb
- it is difficult to maintain positioning of the hindlimbs and the patellas often are noted to have shifted laterally on this view
- remove tail from radiation field
- in a nondysplastic dog, subluxation of the femoral heads laterally will not be attainable

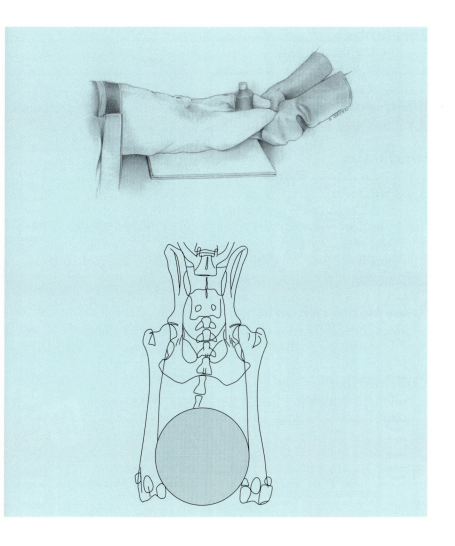

Hip dysplasia study – ventrodorsal view using a stressed half-axial view

Body
- place in dorsal recumbency on pad or in trough
- use a thoracoabdominal compression band
- palpate sternum (xyphoid process) on midline to insure correct position

Forelimbs
- extend limbs cranially
- place sandbags across forelimbs

Head and neck
- extend head in natural position

Hindlimbs
- place cassette in position
- extend limbs
  - hold hocks with gloved hands
  - position tibias parallel to each other and parallel to the table top
  - flex limbs so femurs are at a 45° angle to the table top
  - force the hindlimbs toward the table top

X-ray beam centering
- direct vertical beam on pelvis between the hip joints
- make exposure at the time of maximum force on hindlimbs

Collimation
- collimate closely to include hip joints
- collimate closely to exclude gloved hands

Comments
- this positioning relaxes the extra-articular support structures and is more sensitive in the demonstration of joint laxity
- try to direct pressure on the hindlimbs equally towards the table top to prevent rotation of the pelvis
- this view may be compared with a routine pelvic positioning that may show secondary bony change more clearly
- (this is based on studies by BADERTSCHER, 1977 and FLÜCKIGER, 1997)

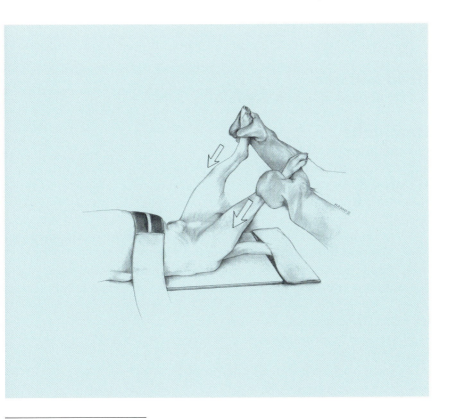

BADERTSCHER R. R. "The half-axial position: Improved radiographic visualization of sublucation in canine hip dysplasia" Thesis – University of Georgia College of Veterinary Medicine 1977.

FLÜCKIGER M. Personal communication 1997.

Hip dysplasia study – ventrodorsal view using a compression-distraction stress method (2 views)

Body
- place in dorsal recumbency on pad or in trough
- use a compression band across thorax
- palpate sternum (xyphoid process) on midline to insure correct position

Forelimbs
- extend limbs cranially
- place sandbags across forelimbs or hold with gloved hands

Head and neck
- extend head in natural position

Hindlimbs
(1) compression view
- place cassette in position
- extend limbs
  - hold hocks with gloved hands
  - flex stifle joints
  - position stifle joints to avoid their superimposition on the hip joints
  - position femurs parallel to each other
  - flex limbs so femurs are at a 90° angle to the table top
  - place a medially directed compressive force on the hips

(2) distraction view
- place cassette in position
- extend limbs
  - hold hocks with gloved hands
  - flex stifle joints
  - position stifle joints to avoid their superimposition on the hip joints
  - position femurs parallel to each other
  - flex limbs so femurs are at a 90° angle to the table top
  - to achieve distraction, place a custom-designed adjustable distracter device between the limbs

X-ray beam centering
- direct vertical beam on pelvis between the hip joints
- for distraction view, make exposure at the time of maximum force on the pelvis

Collimation
- collimate closely to include hip joints
- collimate closely to exclude gloved hands

Comments
- compare the two views to determine the degree of subluxation of the femoral heads
- try to place pressure on the pelvis equally, to prevent rotation of the pelvis
- these views should be compared with a routine pelvic positioning that may show secondary bony change more clearly
- this is based on a study by SMITH et al 1990
- this technique is also referred to as the "Penn Hip Distraction Method"

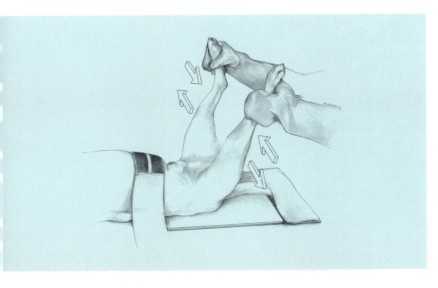

SMITH GK, BIERY DN, GREGOR TP. New concepts of coxofemoral joint stability and the development of a clinical stress-radiographic method for quantitating hip joint laxity in the dog. JAVMA 196: 59–70,1990.

Notes

Forelimb

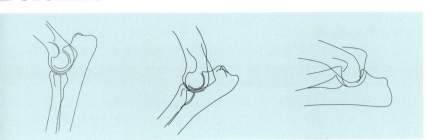

Forelimb

Introduction
- examinations of the forelimb are made to search for many diseases, ranging from those that are congenital/developmental to those that are of traumatic origin
- the character of the bones that make up the forelimb varies widely from the easily positioned long bones of the large and giant breeds to the short, twisted bones of the chondrodystrophoid breeds that are difficult to position

Patient preparation
- inspect haircoat for matted hair, debris, or foreign bodies

Sedation or anesthesia
- not required for most studies

Views
- recommended views
  - lateral
  - craniocaudal (dorsopalmar)
- special views
  - oblique views as required
  - stress views may be of value in studies of the
    - shoulder
    - elbow
    - antebrachiocarpal joint
  - horizontal beam

X-ray technique
– medium to low kVp may permit better evaluation of bones

Use of grid
– most studies are performed using a table top technique while a grid is used on studies of the scapula, shoulder, and humerus of large and giant breeds

Problems in quality of study
– often difficult to position the bones in the proximal part of the limb so they are parallel to the table top for a craniocaudal view
– value of horizontal beam radiography needs be recognized, especially in traumatized patients
– views of the opposite limb are recommended in puppies up to 9 to 12 months of age, so that the appearance of growth centers can be compared in both limbs

Scapula

Introduction
- examinations of the scapula are usually limited to trauma patients plus the uncommon patient with an inflammatory or neoplastic lesion
- the character and location of the scapula makes it difficult to position for radiographic evaluation
- evaluation of the glenoid cavity is better achieved in a study of the shoulder

Patient preparation
- inspect haircoat for matted hair, debris, or foreign bodies

Sedation or anesthesia
- not required for most studies

Views
- recommended views
  - lateral
    - neutral position
    - in dorsal displacement
  - ventrodorsal
- special views
  - oblique views can be made as required

X-ray technique
– medium to low kVp may permit better evaluation of bone

Use of grid
– studies in medium, large, and giant breeds require use of a grid

Comments
– often difficult to position the body part for evaluation, especially in a traumatized patient
– lateral views result in superimposition of the scapulae, creating difficulty in evaluation
– it is possible to make a lateral view with the limb displaced proximally

Scapula – lateral view – neutral position

Body
- place in lateral recumbency on side to be studied
- use a compression band over abdomen

Hindlimbs
- place limbs in a neutral position
- place sandbags over limbs

Head and neck
- place head in neutral position
- place sandbag over neck

Forelimbs
- place cassette on table
- place affected limb next to table top
- displace upper limb caudally as far as possible
  - place sandbag over limb or use tie-down rope
- extend dependent limb cranially
  - place sandbag across dependent limb or use tie-down rope

X-ray beam centering
- direct vertical beam dorsal to shoulder

Collimation
- include both scapulae

Comments
- possible to make study with affected limb uppermost
- possible to make a second study by reversing the positioning of the forelimbs, with the affected limb caudal and the unaffected limb cranial

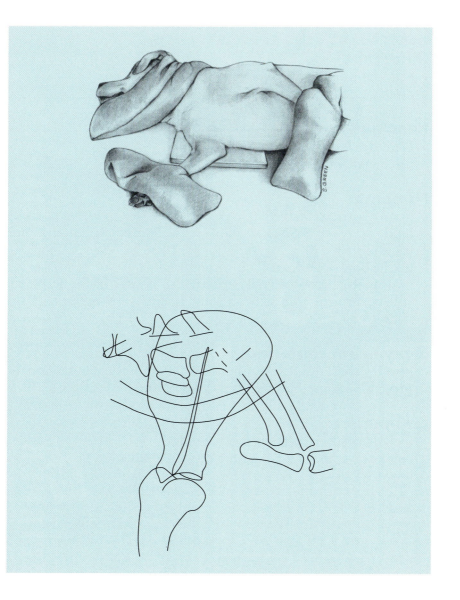

Scapula – lateral view in dorsal displacement

Body
- place in lateral recumbency on side to be studied
- use a compression band over abdomen

Hindlimbs
- place limbs in a neutral position
- place sandbags over limbs

Head and neck
- place head in neutral position
- place sandbag over neck

Forelimbs
- place cassette on table
- hold foot of unaffected limb with gloved hand and pull caudodistally
- hold elbow of affected limb with gloved hand
- push limb dorsoproximally until dorsal border of the scapula is seen to protrude dorsally, causing an abnormal bump over the back

X-ray beam centering
- direct vertical beam dorsal and cranial to thorax, centering on the protrusion caused by the displaced scapula

Collimation
- include displaced scapula and shoulder
- collimate so gloved hands are not within radiation field

Comments
– excellent technique for study of the body of the scapula
– painful to use in a dog with a fracture
– may require sedation or anesthesia

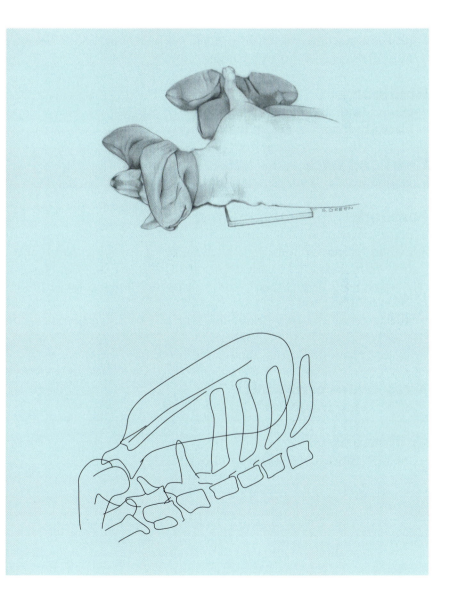

Scapula – caudocranial (ventrodorsal) view

Body
- place in dorsal recumbency on pad or in trough
- use a compression band across abdomen
- position sternum (xyphoid process) approximately 30° laterally away from the limb to be studied

Hindlimbs
- extend caudally in neutral position
- place sandbags across hindlimbs

Head and neck
- extend head in natural position

Forelimbs
- place cassette on table top
- extend affected limb as far cranially as possible until ante-brachium is parallel to table top
  - place sandbag across forelimb or use tie-down rope or hold in gloved hand
- unaffected limb is positioned in a neutral position adjacent to the thorax
  - place sandbag across unaffected forelimb

X-ray beam centering
- direct beam at scapula

Collimation
- include entire scapula and shoulder

Comments
- palpate scapula and determine that the blade is positioned perpendicular to the table top and displaced laterally away from the ribs
- this positioning with the limb fully extended may be painful in many patients

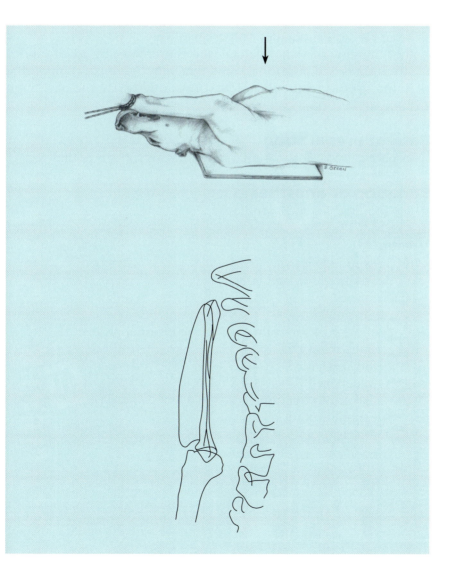

Shoulder

Introduction
– examinations of the shoulder are most commonly performed to identify congenital/developmental lesions (osteochondrosis of the humeral head) or tumors of the proximal humerus (osteosarcomas)
– often this study includes only a lateral view
– the limitation of a single lateral view is overcome by use of various stress views and positional views that alter the relationship of the humeral head to the glenoid cavity and illustrate the maximum range of motion within the joint

Patient preparation
– inspect haircoat for matted hair, debris, or foreign bodies

Sedation or anesthesia
– not required for most studies

Views
– recommended views
  – neutrally positioned lateral
– special views
  – caudocranial
  – craniocaudal for evaluation of the bicipital groove
  – lateral stress views
    – fully extended
    – fully flexed
    – maximum traction
    – external rotation (supination)
    – internal rotation (pronation)

X-ray technique
– medium to low kVp may permit better evaluation of bone

Use of grid
– most studies are performed using a table top method, while a grid is needed on studies of the shoulder of large and giant breeds

Comments
– difficult to position for the caudocranial view
– views of the opposite limb are recommended in puppies up to 9 to 12 months of age so that the appearance of growth centers can be compared in both limbs

Shoulder – lateral view in neutral position

Body
- place in lateral recumbency on side to be studied
- use a compression band over abdomen

Hindlimbs
- place limbs in neutral position
- place sandbags over limbs

Head and neck
- place head in hyperextended position
- place sandbag over neck

Forelimbs
- place cassette on table top
- remove upper limb from field by caudal displacement
  - hold limb with sandbag, tie-down rope, or gloved hand
- extend the affected limb cranially
  - hold limb with sandbag or tie-down rope or gloved hand

X-ray beam centering
- direct vertical beam on shoulder

Collimation
- include glenoid cavity, shoulder, and proximal humerus
- may include entire scapula

Comments

- insure that shoulder is ventral to the trachea
- avoid rotating body, with resulting elevation of sternum from table top, because this results in obliquity of the shoulder joint

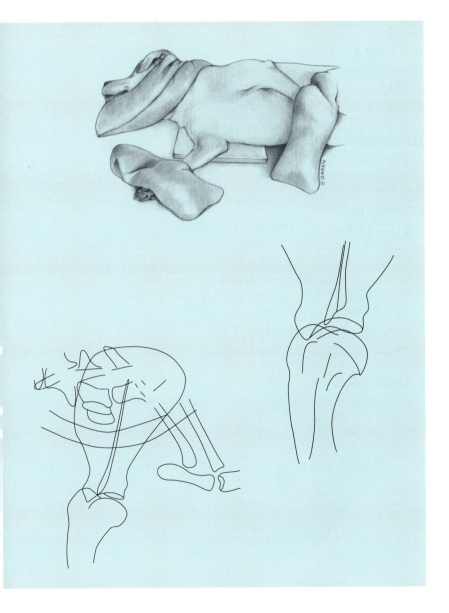

Shoulder – lateral view in stressed positions

Body
- place in lateral recumbency on side to be studied
- use a compression band over abdomen

Hindlimbs
- place limb in neutral position
- place sandbags over limbs

Head and neck
- place head in hyperextended position
- place sandbag over neck

Forelimbs
- place cassette on table top
- remove upper limb from field by caudal displacement
  - hold limb with sandbag, tie-down rope, or gloved hand
- position the affected limb (see figures)
  - hold limb with sandbag or tie-down rope or gloved hand

X-ray beam centering
- direct vertical beam on shoulder

Collimation
- include glenoid cavity, shoulder, and proximal humerus

Comments

– views include those made with the limb in maximum (see drawings below)
  – flexion
  – extension
  – traction
  – internal rotation
  – external rotation
– insure that shoulder joint is ventral to trachea
– avoid rotating body, with resulting elevation of sternum away from the table top, because this results in obliquity of the joint

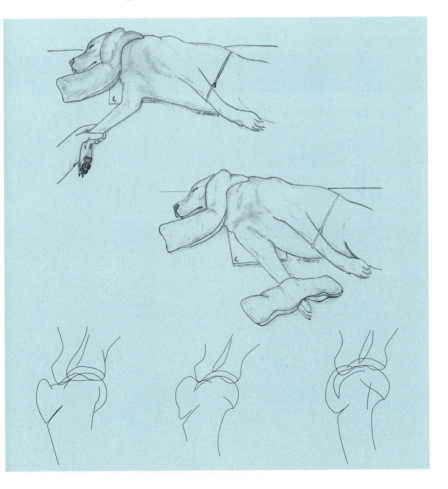

Shoulder – caudocranial (ventrodorsal) view

Body
- place in dorsal recumbency on pad or in trough
- use a compression band across abdomen
- position sternum (xyphoid process) away from the affected limb

Hindlimbs
- extend caudally in neutral position
- place sandbags across hindlimbs

Head and neck
- extend head in natural position

Forelimbs
- place the unaffected limb in a neutral position adjacent to the ribs
- place cassette on table top
- extend affected limb cranially
- place antebrachium parallel to table top
    - place sandbag across forelimb or use tie-down rope or hold in gloved hand

X-ray beam centering
- direct beam at shoulder

Collimation
- include glenoid cavity, shoulder, and proximal humerus

Comments
- palpate scapula and determine that it is positioned perpendicular to the table top
- this positioning with the limb fully extended may be painful
- it is possible to position forelimb in supination or pronation to alter positioning (see drawings below)

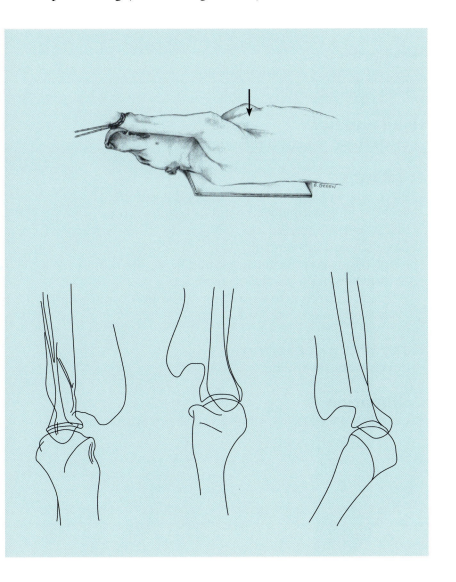

Shoulder – craniocaudal view

Body
- place in dorsal recumbency on pad or in trough
- use a compression band across abdomen
- position sternum (xyphoid process) approximately 30° laterally away from the affected limb

Hindlimbs
- extend caudally in neutral position
- place sandbags across hindlimbs

Head and neck
- extend head in natural position

Forelimbs
- place unaffected limb in an extended position
    - hold limb with gloved hand or tie-down rope
- place cassette on table top
- flex affected limb caudally
    - place adjacent to, but separated from, the thoracic wall
    - place humerus parallel to table top
    - place sandbag across forelimb or use tie-down rope or hold in gloved hand

X-ray beam centering
- direct beam at shoulder

Collimation
- include glenoid cavity, shoulder, and proximal humerus

Comments

– this view permits evaluation of the bicipital groove
– palpate the scapula and determine that it is positioned perpendicular to the table top

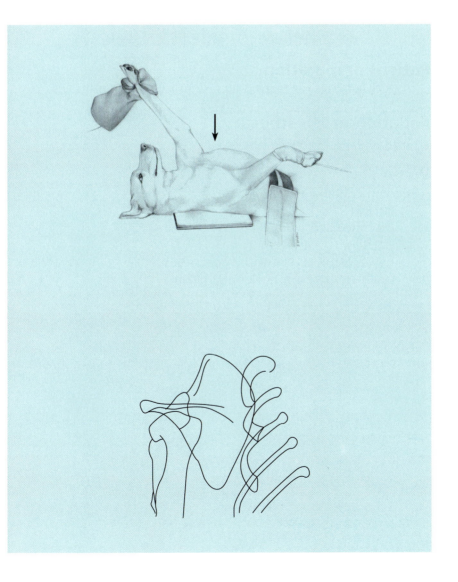

Humerus

Introduction
- examination of the humerus is required most commonly in trauma patients
- the lateral view is made easily while the craniocaudal or caudocranial view requires positioning that is difficult to achieve
- use of a horizontal beam is stressed for this study

Patient preparation
- inspect haircoat for matted hair, debris, or foreign bodies

Sedation or anesthesia
- not required for most studies

Views
- recommended views
  - lateral
  - extended craniocaudal
- special views
  - flexed craniocaudal with vertical beam
  - caudocranial with horizontal beam

X-ray technique
– medium to low kVp may permit better evaluation of bone

Use of grid
– most studies are performed using a table top method, while a grid is required on studies in large and giant breeds

Comments
– difficult to position for the craniocaudal or caudocranial view
– views of the opposite limb are recommended in puppies up to 9 to 12 months of age so that the appearance of growth centers can be compared in both limbs

Humerus – lateral view

Body
– place in lateral recumbency with limb to be studied dependent
– use a compression band over abdomen

Hindlimbs
– place limbs in neutral position
– place sandbags over limbs

Head and neck
– place head in neutral position
– place sandbag over neck

Forelimbs
– remove upper limb from field, displacing it caudally with the shoulder fully flexed
  – hold limb with tie-down rope or sandbag
– place cassette on table top
– extend the affected limb cranially with elbow partially flexed
  – hold limb with sandbag or tie-down rope or gloved hand

X-ray beam centering
– direct vertical beam on midshaft of humerus

Collimation
– include shoulder, humerus, and elbow

Comments
– insure that shoulder joint is ventral to the trachea
– consider which portion of the humerus is most important and adjust exposure for that tissue thickness
– the shoulder is underexposured or the elbow is overexposed in most radiographs because of the great difference in tissue thickness

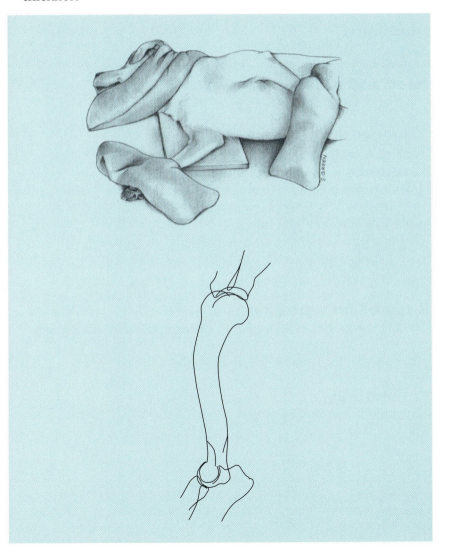

Humerus – craniocaudal view with limb extended

Body
- place in sternal recumbency on pad or in trough
- use a compression band across the back

Hindlimbs
- extend caudally in neutral position

Head and neck
- hyperextend head laterally away from the affected limb
- may need gloved hand to hold head hyperextended to remove it from radiation field

Forelimbs
- place unaffected limb in an extended position
  - place sandbag across forelimb
- place cassette on table top
- extend affected limb as far cranially and distally as possible
  - place sandbag across forelimb or use tie-down rope or use gloved hand

X-ray beam centering
- angle X-ray beam 10° to 20° distoproximally (craniocaudally) from the vertical
- center the beam at the midshaft of the humerus

Collimation
- include humerus and elbow

Comments
– this view does not permit evaluation of the proximal humerus but is the quickest and easiest way to obtain a view of the midshaft and distal humerus
– note that this positioning does not place the humerus parallel to the table top, thus distortion of the bone is present
– this positioning with the limb fully extended may be painful in a trauma case

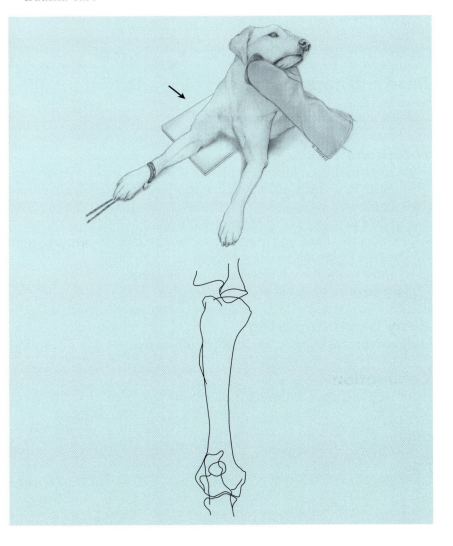

Humerus – craniocaudal view with limb flexed

Body
– place in dorsal recumbency on pad or in trough
– place compression band across abdomen

Hindlimbs
– place in frog-leg position
– place sandbags across hindlimbs

Head and neck
– extend head
– place sandbags lateral to head

Forelimbs
– extend unaffected limb
    – hold limb in position with a tie-down line or with gloved hand, or
    – place sandbag across unaffected limb
– flex affected limb and position as far caudally as possible until humerus is parallel to the table top
    – use tie-down rope or hold in gloved hand
– place cassette beneath body

X-ray beam centering
– direct vertical beam at midshaft of humerus

Collimation
– include shoulder, humerus, and elbow

Comments
– this view provides the best study of the humerus, using a positioning that is rather easy for both patient and technician
– this view is the least painful because it does not require full extension of the limb
– object-film distance is increased causing magnification
– magnification is uniform since humerus is parallel to the table top

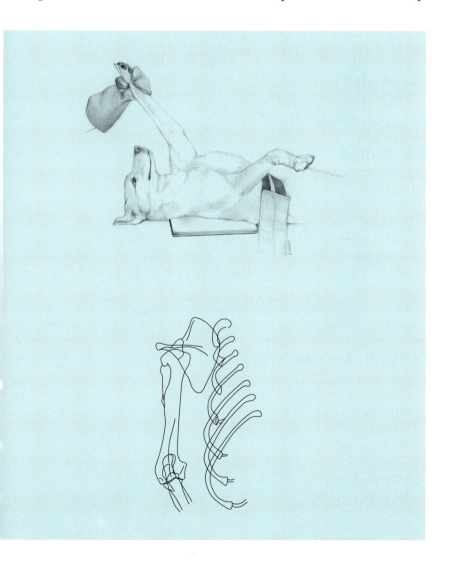

Humerus – caudocranial view with horizontal beam

Body
– place in lateral recumbency on pad, with affected limb uppermost

Hindlimbs
– extend caudally in neutral position
– place sandbags across limbs

Head and neck
– place head in neutral position
– place sandbags across the neck

Forelimbs
– place affected limb on a sponge block so humerus is parallel to the table top
– extend affected limb
– use tie-down rope or gloved hand to extend limb
– place cassette vertical to the table top against cranial aspect of humerus
– use sandbag or positioning device to hold cassette in vertical position
– place unaffected limb in neutral position
– place sandbag across unaffected limb or use tie-down rope

X-ray beam centering
– position the X-ray tube caudally
– direct the beam in a horizontal position in a caudal to cranial direction
– center the beam at the midshaft of the humerus perpendicular to the cassette

Collimation
– include shoulder, humerus, and elbow

Comments
– this view provides a good study of the humerus but requires extensive repositioning of the X-ray tube
– positioning for this view is the least painful for the dog because it does not require full extension of the limb
– object-film distance is slightly increased but since the humerus is parallel to the cassette the magnification is uniform

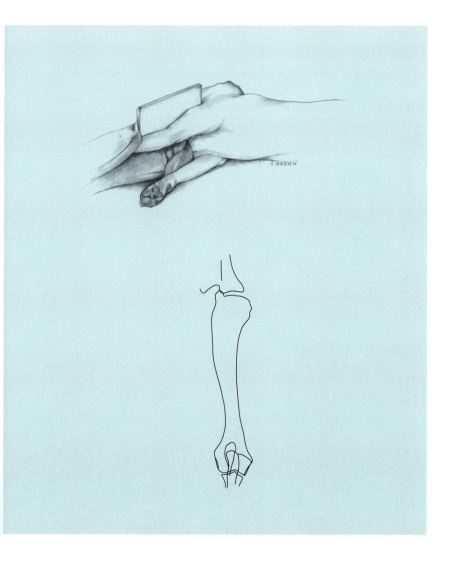

Elbow

Introduction
– examinations of the elbow are most commonly performed to identify developmental disease or in trauma patients
– lateral views are made easily, while craniocaudal views are more difficult to make and to evaluate
– views made with a horizontal beam are more diagnostic

Patient preparation
– inspect haircoat for matted hair, debris, or foreign bodies

Sedation or anesthesia
– not required for most studies

Views
– recommended views
    – lateral
    – craniocaudal
– special views
    – lateral
        – flexed
        – extended
    – oblique
    – craniocaudal with a horizontal beam

X-ray technique
– medium to low kVp may permit better evaluation of bone

Use of grid
– studies are performed using a table top method without a grid

Comments

- it is difficult to position the tube for the craniocaudal view made with a vertical beam
- views of the opposite limb are recommended in puppies up to 9 to 12 months of age so that the appearance of growth centers can be compared in both limbs
- study in short-legged dogs is particularly difficult
- may be helpful to angle the beam craniocaudally

Elbow – lateral view

Body
- place in lateral recumbency on side to be studied
- use a compression band over abdomen

Hindlimbs
- place limbs in neutral position
- place sandbags over limbs

Head and neck
- place head in neutral position
- place sandbag over neck

Forelimbs
- remove upper limb from field by displacing caudally with shoulder fully flexed
- hold limb with tie-down rope or sandbag
- place cassette on table top
- position the affected limb cranially with elbow partially flexed (120° extension)
- place elbow on cassette
- hold limb with sandbag or tie-down rope

X-ray beam centering
- direct vertical beam on the elbow

Collimation
- include distal humerus, elbow, and proximal radius and ulna

Comments

- by having the limb partially flexed it is possible to avoid unintentional supination or pronation of the foot that will affect the appearance of the radius and ulna
- placing the limb in greater extension (>120°) allows for better evaluation of joint congruity (see drawings below)
- placing the limb in near complete flexion (<45°) allows for more complete evaluation of the anconeal process (see drawings below)

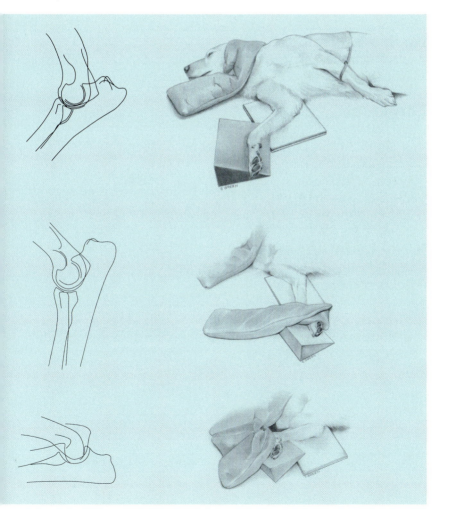

Elbow – craniocaudal view with vertical beam

Body
- place in sternal recumbency
- use a compression band over back

Hindlimbs
- place limbs in neutral position

Head and neck
- place head in hyperextended position
- use gloved hand to displace the head laterally

Forelimbs
- partially extend unaffected limb
    - hold limb with tie-down rope or sandbag
- place cassette on table top
- extend affected limb as completely as possible
- place elbow on cassette
- hold limb with tie-down rope or sandbag or gloved hand

X-ray beam centering
- angle beam 10° to 20 ° craniocaudally
- center beam on elbow

Collimation
- include distal humerus, elbow, and proximal radius and ulna

Comments

– view requires that the limb be placed in as complete extension as possible
– tension on the limb may be painful and may require use of a gloved hand to maintain position
– rotate the limb internally or externally to make oblique views for better evaluation of lateral and medial coronoid processes and distal humerus (see drawings below)

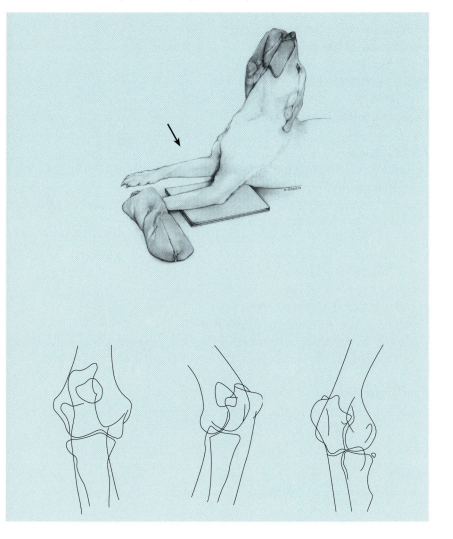

Elbow – craniocaudal view with horizontal beam

Body
- place in lateral recumbency with affected limb uppermost
- use compression band over thorax

Hindlimbs
- place limbs in neutral position
- place sandbags over limbs

Head and neck
- place head in neutral or hyperextended position
- place sandbag over neck

Forelimbs
- extend unaffected limb in neutral position
- hold limb with tie-down rope or sandbag
- place affected limb on sponge block so limb is parallel to table top
- extend affected limb as completely as possible
- hold limb with tie-down rope or sandbag or gloved hand
- place vertically oriented cassette on table top caudal to elbow
- place sandbag behind cassette

X-ray beam centering
- position the X-ray tube cranially
- direct the beam in a horizontal plane in a craniocaudal direction
- center the beam on the elbow perpendicular to the cassette

Collimation
- include distal humerus, elbow, and proximal radius and ulna

Comments

- this view provides an excellent view of the extended elbow but requires repositioning of the X-ray tube
- this view is the least painful because it does not require the dog to bear weight on the forelimb
- it may be difficult to determine the exact positioning of the tube because of the variance in positioning of the shoulder joint
- this positioning is relatively easy in an awake dog

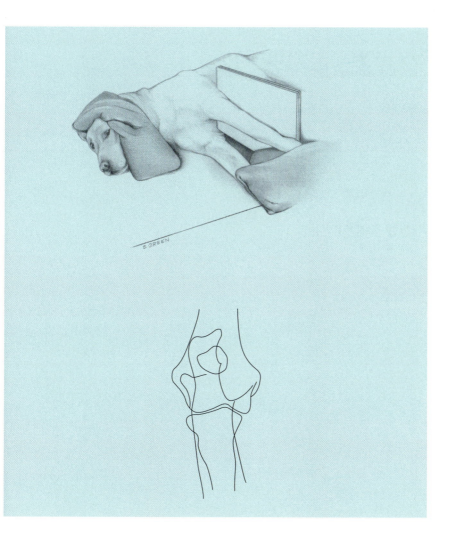

Antebrachium

Introduction
– examinations of the more distal parts of the forelimb are relatively easy to perform because of a greater ease in positioning and only a minimal soft tissue thickness

Patient preparation
– inspect haircoat for matted hair, debris, or foreign bodies

Sedation or anesthesia
– not required for most studies

Views
– recommended views
  – lateral
  – craniocaudal
– special views
  – oblique

X-ray technique
– medium to low kVp may permit better evaluation of bone

Use of grid
– studies are performed using a table top method without a grid

Comments
– in dogs with growth abnormalities or malunion fractures, the foot can be placed in an anatomically correct position, artificially correcting a defect of rotation or angulation

Antebrachium – lateral view

Body
- place in lateral recumbency on side to be studied
- use compression band over abdomen

Hindlimbs
- place limbs in neutral position
- place sandbags over limbs

Head and neck
- place head in neutral position
- place sandbag over neck

Forelimbs
- remove upper limb from field by displacecaudally with shoulder fully flexed
- hold limb with tie-down rope or sandbag
- place cassette on table top
- place antebrachium on cassette
- position the affected limb partially extended
- hold limb with sandbag or tie-down rope or gloved hand

X-ray beam centering
- direct vertical beam on the middle portion of the antebrachium

Collimation
- include elbow, radius and ulna, and antebrachiocarpal joint

Comments
- by having the elbow partially flexed it is possible to avoid supination or pronation of the foot affecting the manner in which the radius and ulna are projected on the radiograph
- may use a large cassette divided in half with a lead sheet or use collimator to place lateral and craniocaudal views on the radiograph

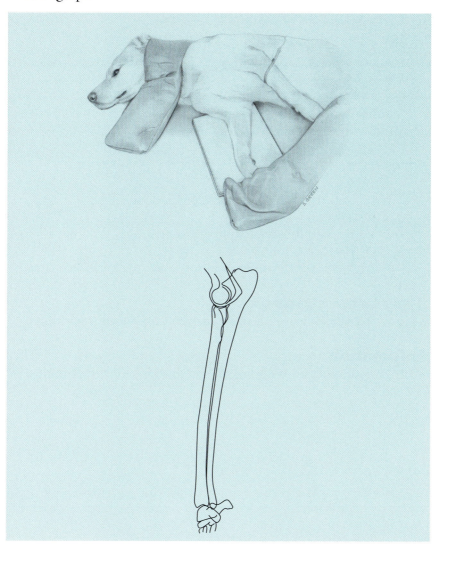

Antebrachium – craniocaudal view with vertical beam

Body
- place in sternal recumbency
- use compression band over back

Hindlimbs
- place limbs in neutral position
- place sandbags over limbs

Head and neck
- place head in hyperextended position
- use gloved hand to displace the head laterally

Forelimbs
- extend unaffected limb in a neutral position
    - hold limb with tie-down rope or sandbag
- place cassette on table top
- extend affected limb as completely as possible
- place antebrachium on cassette
    - hold limb with tie-down rope or sandbag or gloved hand

X-ray beam centering
- direct a vertical beam on the midshaft of the radius and ulna

Collimation
- include elbow, radius and ulna, and antebrachiocarpal joint

Comments

– place a sandbag just caudal to the elbow to prevent the dog from
  withdrawing the limb

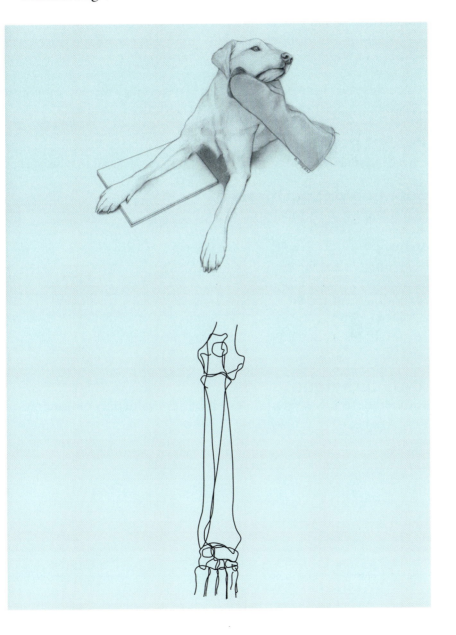

Carpus, Metacarpus, and Digits

Introduction
- examinations of the feet are relatively easy to perform because of the ease in positioning and only a minimal soft tissue thickness
- stress radiography is useful in determining the extent of joint laxity
- use of positioning devices such as woodens spoon or plastic paddle to position the foot for stress studies is helpful

Patient preparation
- inspect haircoat for matted hair, debris, or foreign bodies

Sedation or anesthesia
- not required for most studies

Views
- recommended views
    - lateral
    - dorsopalmar
- special views
    - oblique
    - stress

X-ray technique
- medium to low kVp may permit better evaluation of bone

Use of grid
– studies are performed using a table top method without a grid

Comments
– techniques are similar for radiography of all parts of the foot
– views of the opposite limb are recommended in puppies up to 9 to 12 months of age so that the appearance of growth centers can be compared in both limbs
– it is possible to tie gauze around a foot to enhance positioning
– the distal interphalangeal joint is normally hyperflexed, requiring use of a compression device to flatten the digit against the film to permit evaluation of the joint spaces on dorsopalmar views
– it is relatively easy to obtain two oblique views and place all four views of the foot on a single radiograph

Carpus, metacarpus, and digits – lateral view

Body
- place in lateral recumbency on side to be studied
- place a compression band over abdomen

Hindlimbs
- place limbs in neutral position
- place sandbags over limbs

Head and neck
- place head in neutral position
- place sandbag over neck

Forelimbs
- remove upper limb from field by displace caudaly with shoulder flexed
  - hold limb with tie-down rope or sandbag
- place cassette on table top
- position the affected limb cranially in a neutral position
- place foot on cassette
  - hold limb with sandbag or tie-down rope or gloved hand
- use a positioning device to control position of the foot
- make additional views after positioning the foot on cassette using a spoon or paddle
  - hyperflexed
  - hyperextended

X-ray beam centering
- direct vertical beam on the foot

Collimation
- include distal radius and ulna, carpus, metacarpus, and digits

Comments

- by having the elbow partially flexed it is possible to avoid supination or pronation of the foot affecting the appearance of the foot on the radiograph
- use positioning device to create hyperextension on hyperflexion views
- can hold positioning device with sandbags
- can use a gauze strip to position a digit in a hyperextended position so that it is not covered by the other digits

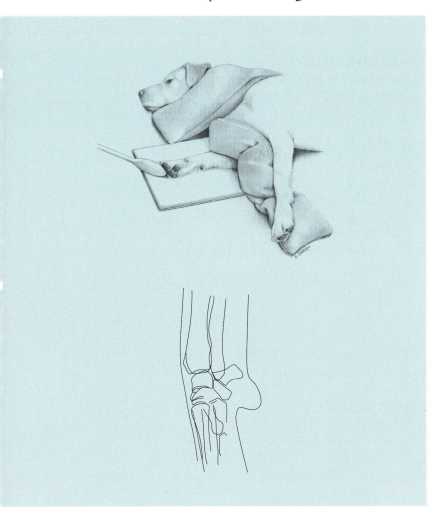

Carpus, metacarpus, and digits – dorsopalmar view

Body
– place in sternal recumbency
– use a compression band over back

Hindlimbs
– place limbs in neutral position
– place sandbags over limbs

Head and neck
– place head in hyperextended position or turn head laterally away from the limb to be studied
– use gloved hand or sandbag to position the head

Forelimbs
– extend unaffected limb
    – hold limb with tie-down rope or sandbag
– place cassette on table top
– extend affected limb as completely as possible
– place foot on cassette
– use tie-down rope around distal antebrachium to maintain limb extension
– place in neutral, axially (medially) stressed, or abaxially (laterally) stressed position
– use positioning device to create stressed position

X-ray beam centering
– direct a vertical beam on the foot

Collimation
– include carpus, metacarpus, and digits

Comments
– place a sandbag just caudal to the elbow to prevent the dog from withdrawing the limb

– positioning devices are of great value in creating pressure in an axial or abaxial direction for the stress views
– can use sandbag to hold handle of positioning device
– use a plastic paddle to force the foot in the neutral position against the cassette to create full extension of the metacarpo-phalangeal and inter-phalangeal joints
– use positioning to make medial and lateral oblique views (see drawings below)

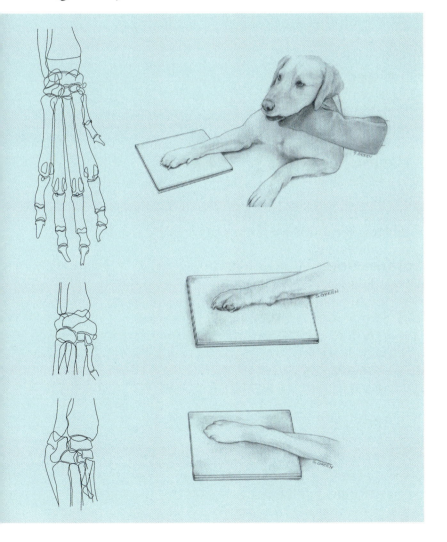

Digits – lateral view

Body
- place in lateral recumbency on the side to be studied
- use a compression band over abdomen

Head and neck
- place head in neutral position
- place sandbag over neck

Hindlimbs
- place sandbags over limbs

Forelimbs
- remove upper limb from field by lateral displacement
  - hold limb with tie-down rope or sandbag
- position the affected foot on the cassette
- extend the limb

X-ray beam centering
- direct vertical beam on the digits

Collimation
- include digits

Comments

– the affected digit can be separated for radiography (see drawing below)
  – place gauze around the unaffected digits and pull in a palmar direction
  – place gauze around the affected digit and pull in a dorsal direction
  – separate the digit by pulling on both gauze strips
  – fasten gauze to the edge of the table or wrap around a sandbag
– it is also possible to obtain near-lateral views of a digit by tilting the foot slightly

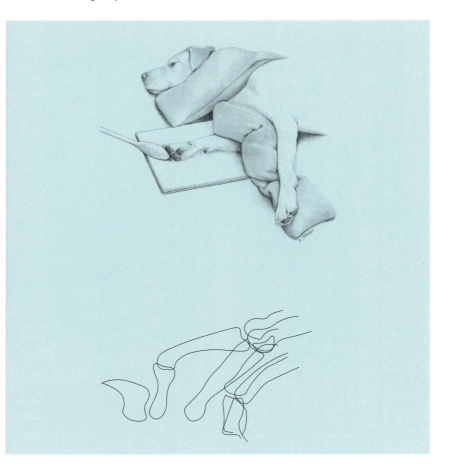

Notes

Hindlimb

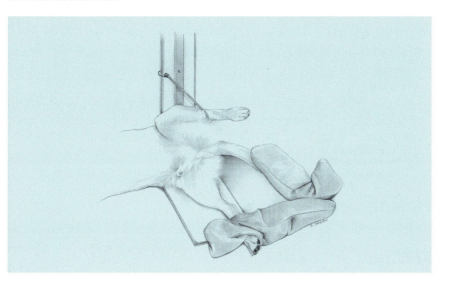

Hindlimb

Introduction
- examinations of the pelvic limb are made to search for many diseases, ranging from those that are congenital/developmental to those that are traumatic
- the character of the bones that make up the pelvic limb varies widely from the more easily positioned long bones of the large and giant breeds to the short, twisted bones of the chondro-dystrophoid breeds that are difficult to position
- discussion of the hip joint is included in studies of the pelvis

Patient preparation
- inspect haircoat for matted hair, debris, or foreign bodies

Sedation or anesthesia
- not required for most studies

Views
- recommended views
  - lateral
  - craniocaudal
- special views
  - oblique views as required
  - stress views are of value in studies of the
    - stifle
    - tibiotarsal (talocrural) joint

X-ray technique
– medium to low kVp may permit better evaluation of bone

Use of grid
– most studies are performed using a table top method, while a grid is used on studies of the femur of medium, large, and giant breeds

Comments
– it is often difficult to position the femur parallel to the table top for the craniocaudal or caudocranial views
– the value of horizontal beam radiography needs to be recognized
– views of the opposite limb in puppies up to 9 to 12 months permit a comparison of growth centers

Femur

Introduction
- examinations of the femur usually follow trauma
- evaluation of the proximal femur and the hip joint is included in the examination of the pelvis

Patient preparation
- inspect haircoat for matted hair, debris, or foreign bodies

Sedation or anesthesia
- not required for most studies

Views
- recommended views
  - lateral view
  - craniocaudal view using vertical beam
- special views
  - caudocranial view using horizontal beam
  - ventrodorsal view with limb in a fully flexed position ("frog-leg")

X-ray exposure
- medium to low kVp may permit better evaluation of bone

Use of grid
- studies in medium, large, and giant breeds require use of a grid

Comments
- because it is difficult to position the femur so it is parallel to the table top when making a craniocaudal view using a vertical beam, it is often helpful to sit dog up on rump to achieve adequate positioning
- value of horizontal beam radiography needs to be recognized
- views of the opposite limb in puppies up to 9 to 12 months provide an opportunity for comparison of growth centers

Femur – lateral view

Body
- place in lateral recumbency on side to be studied
- use a compression band over thorax

Head and neck
- place head in neutral position
- place sandbag over neck

Forelimbs
- place forelimbs in neutral position
- hold limbs with sandbags

Hindlimbs
- unaffected hindlimb is abducted and removed from radiation field
    - use tie-down rope to tie limb in position
- place cassette on table top
- affected limb is extended, with stifle joint remaining partially flexed
    - hold limb with sandbag over foot or use tie-down rope or use a gloved hand

X-ray beam centering
- direct vertical beam on midshaft of femur

Collimation
- include coxofemoral joint, femur, and stifle

Comments
– it is possible to angle the X-ray beam distoproximally if the upper limb cannot be completely removed from the radiation field
– usually the proximal femur is underexposed
– may need to position prepuce and penis out of the radiation field
– it is possible to position a fluid-filled plastic bag (fluid therapy bag) around the limb to equal out the difference in tissue thickness

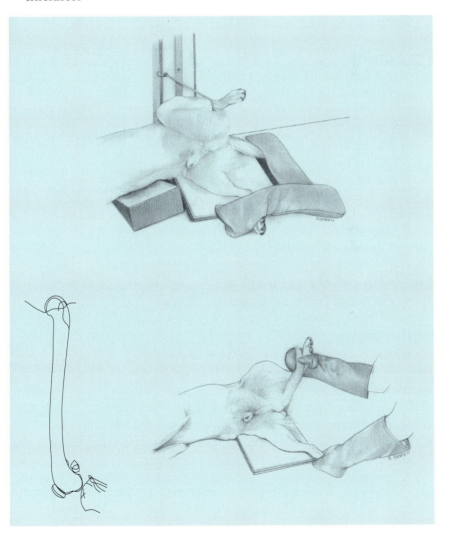

Femur – lateral view (alternative view)

Body
- place in lateral recumbency on side to be studied
- use a compression band over abdomen

Head and neck
- place head in neutral position
- place sandbag over neck

Forelimbs
- place forelimbs in neutral position
- hold limbs with sandbags

Hindlimbs
- unaffected hindlimb
  - limb is partially extended
  - use sandbag or tie-down rope to position limb
- place cassette on table top
- position affected limb adjacent to the ventral abdomen
  - extend hip joint fully stifle joint with partially flexed
- hold limb with sandbag over foot or use tie-down rope

X-ray beam centering
- direct vertical beam on midshaft of femur

Collimation
- include coxofemoral joint, femur, and stifle

Comments
- this view is helpful in examining a fractured femur in instances where patient manipulation needs to be minimal
- this position leaves the dog in a more neutral position that may be more comfortable to the dog

- the soft tissues of the abdomen "wrap around" the proximal limb creating a soft tissue density that is uniform throughout the length of the femur and that permits visualization of the entire femur
- abdominal tissues may contain both air and radiodense material, creating artifacts that may be superimposed over the femur being studied
- the femur to be examined is under the caudoventral portion of the abdomen and may have the prepuce and penis superimposed
- the study is of value in the traumatized patient where extensive positioning of the pelvic limbs is contraindicated
- the hip joint may be covered by the opposite hip joint and poorly demonstrated

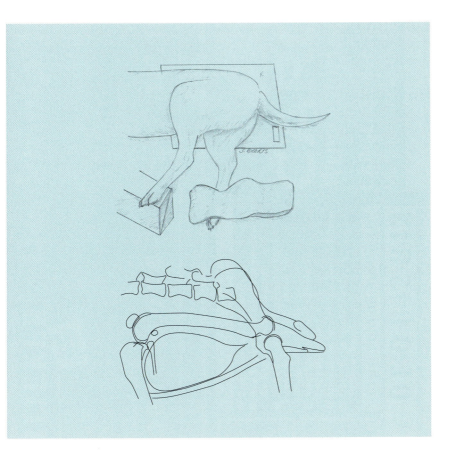

Femur – craniocaudal view with limb extended

Body
– place in dorsal recumbency on pad or in trough
– use compression band across cranial abdomen
– rotate the body slightly
– place a sponge under the pelvis on the affected side to cause elevation of the pelvis

Head and neck
– extend head in neutral position

Forelimbs
– extend limbs beside head
– place sandbags across forelimbs

Hindlimbs
– place cassette on table top
– extend limbs caudally in neutral position
– position both limbs in same manner
– place sandbags across hindlimbs or use tie-down rope or use gloved hands

X-ray beam centering
– direct vertical beam at midshaft of femur

Collimation
– include coxofemoral joint, femur, and stifle

Comments
- this is the most common view used to study femoral injury but it is a less successful study because the positioning places the femur at an angle to the table top, thus resulting in shortening of the bone on the radiograph
- this view is stressful and painful to the patient with a femoral fracture or hip joint disease
- it is possible to force the affected limb towards the table top using gloved hands (not recommended because of pain)
- it is often helpful to sit the dog on its rump to achieve adequate positioning
- it is possible to make this view with the limbs in a hyperflexed position ("frog-leg") (p 158)

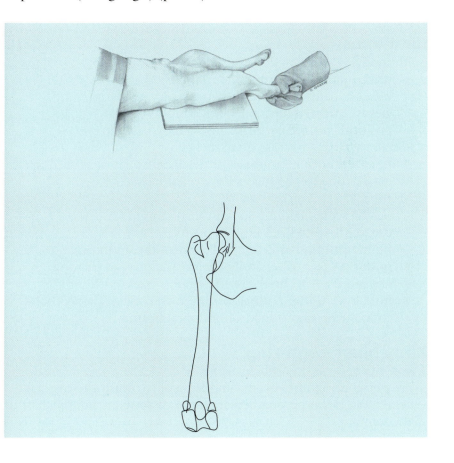

Femur – caudocranial view with horizontal beam

Body
- place in lateral recumbency on pad, with affected limb uppermost

Head and neck
- place head in neutral position
- place sandbag over neck

Forelimbs
- place limbs in neutral position
- place sandbags across forelimbs

Hindlimbs
- Method 1
    - place unaffected limb in neutral position
    - use sandbag to hold limb in position
    - elevate affected limb on sponge block
    - position cassette vertically just cranial to femur
    - use sandbags to hold cassette against limb
    - hold limb using sandbags or tie-down ropes or gloved hand
    - rotate tube to produce a horizontal beam
- Method 2
    - place unaffected limb in neutral position
    - use sandbag to hold limb in position
    - tightly position affected limb against the abdomen
    - position cassette vertically against the back of the dog
    - use sandbags to hold cassette against back
    - hold limb using sandbag or tie-down rope or gloved hand
    - rotate tube to produce a horizontal beam

X-ray beam centering
- reposition the X-ray tube caudally
- direct the horizontal beam caudocranially toward the cassette
- center the beam perpendicular to the cassette at the midshaft of the femur

Collimation
– include femur and stifle

Comments
– either view provides a good study of the femur but requires repositioning of the X-ray tube
– both techniques are less painful than those made with a vertical beam because they do not require extension of the limb
– method 1 does not include the proximal femur because of difficulty in placing the cassette proximally
– method 2 can include the entire femur, but produces increased object-film distance and greater scatter radiation because the limb is tightly placed against the abdomen (see drawings below)

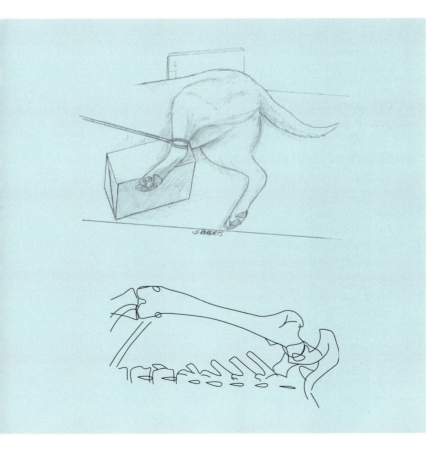

Stifle

Introduction
- an important joint to study in the dog because of injury due to accute trauma and cruciate ligament disease with associated degenerative changes
- all three parts of the joint need to be evaluated, the medial femorotibial, the lateral femorotibial, and the femoropatellar
- special attention may need be given to radiography of the patella
- on the caudocranial view, the degree of limb extension and/or beam angle alters the appearance of the condylar region, ranging from "tunnel" view that provides visualization of the intra-condylar region to a view that projects the more cranial articular portion of the condyles
- the joint can be radiographed in a fully extended position using a horizontal beam
- it is possible to study the joint while weight-bearing mode

Patient preparation
- inspect haircoat for matted hair, debris, or foreign bodies

Sedation or anesthesia
- not required for most studies

Views
- recommended views
  - lateral view
  - caudocranial view using vertical beam
- special views
  - caudocranial view using horizontal beam
  - skyline view of the patella
  - weight-bearing views
  - oblique views

X-ray technique
– medium to low kVp may permit better evaluation of bone

Use of grid
– views do not require use of a grid

Comments
– it is impossible to position the hindlimb so it is fully extended for the caudocranial view with a vertical beam
– the value of horizontal beam radiography is important to understand
– views of the opposite limb are recommended in puppies up to 9 to 12 months of age so that the appearance of growth centers can be compared in both limbs

Stifle – lateral view

Body
- place in lateral recumbency on side to be studied
- use a compression band over abdomen

Head and neck
- place head in neutral position
- place sandbag over neck

Forelimbs
- place forelimbs in neutral position
- hold limbs with sandbags

Hindlimbs
- unaffected hindlimb is abducted and removed from radiation field
  - use tie-down rope to tie limb in position
- place cassette on table top
- place limb on cassette
- affected limb is extended with stifle flexed
  - hold limb with sandbag over foot or use tie-down rope or use gloved hand

X-ray beam centering
- direct vertical beam on stifle

Collimation
- include distal femur, patella, stifle joint, and proximal tibia

Comments

– different degrees of flexion of the joint may be created (see drawings below)
– may need to position prepuce and penis out of the radiation field
– control position of the tail

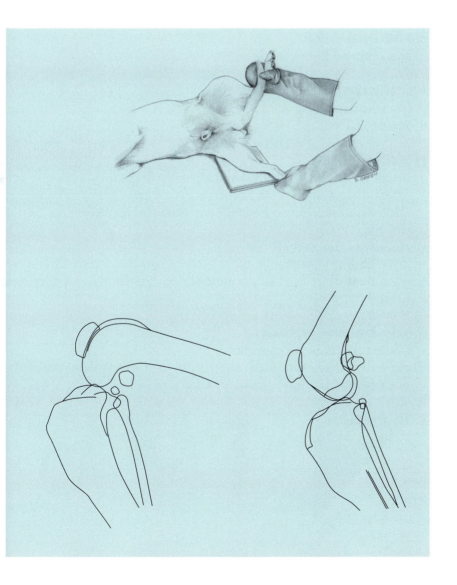

Stifle – caudocranial view

Body
- place in sternal recumbency on pad or in trough
- use sponge to elevate the pelvis on the unaffected side
- use compression band across back

Head and neck
- extend head in neutral position

Forelimbs
- place limbs in extended position
- place sandbags across forelimbs

Hindlimbs
- unaffected limb is elevated and partially flexed
    - sandbag is placed over limb
- affected limb is fully extended, with the patella resting on a small pad for comfort
- place cassette on table top
- place limb on cassette
- place sandbags across hindlimb or use tie-down rope or use gloved hand

X-ray beam centering
- direct vertical beam at stifle
- the beam may be angled 10° to 20° distoproximally, since the limb cannot be fully extended

Collimation
- include distal femur, patella, stifle, and proximal tibia

Comments

- this is the most common view used but it is difficult to achieve good positioning in a large muscular dog
- it may be stressful and painful to rest the limb on the patella
- note that the femur is at an angle to the table top, resulting in shortening of the bone radiographically
- the vertical beam makes an intracondylar "tunnel" view because of the angle of the femur with the table top
- the angled beam shifts the patella distally and closes the intra-condylar "tunnel"

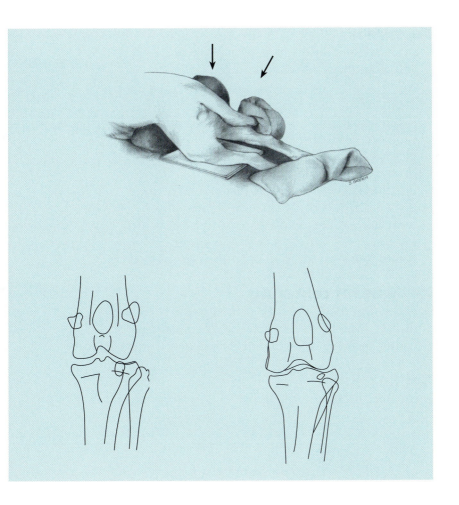

Stifle – caudocranial view with horizontal beam

Body
- place in lateral recumbency on pad, with affected limb uppermost
- use compression band over thorax

Head and neck
- place head in neutral position
- place sandbag over neck

Forelimbs
- place affected limbs in neutral position
- place sandbags across forelimbs

Hindlimbs
- extend unaffected limb in neutral position
  - place sandbag over limb
- elevate affected limb on sponge block
  - fully extend limb
- position cassette vertically just cranial to stifle
- use sandbags to hold cassette against limb
- hold limb using sandbags or use tie-down ropes or use gloved hand
- rotate the X-ray tube to produce a horizontal beam

X-ray beam centering
- reposition the X-ray tube caudally
- direct horizontal beam in a caudocranial direction
- center beam on the stifle perpendicular to the cassette

Collimation
- include distal femur, patella, stifle, and proximal tibia

Comments
- this view provides a good study of the extended stifle but requires repositioning of the X-ray tube
- the technique is less painful because the dog does not support its body weight on the patella or on a painful stifle joint during radiography

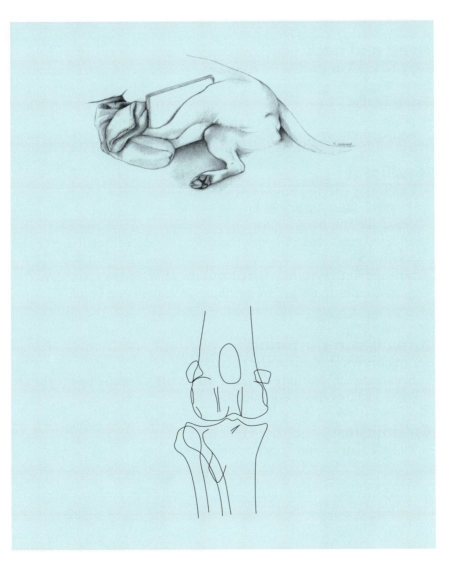

Patella – proximodistal view with limb flexed

Body
- place in sternal recumbency on pad or in trough
- use compression band across back or place sandbags along side of body

Head and neck
- place head in neutral position

Forelimbs
- place limbs in an extended position
- place sandbags across forelimbs

Hindlimbs
- elevate unaffected limb on a sponge block
  - place sandbag across limb
- place cassette on table top
- affected limb is placed with the flexed stifle joint resting on a thin sponge block
- affected limb is tightly flexed and the stifle rests on the cassette
  - place sandbags across hindlimb or use gloved hand
  - sandbags are placed lateral to the limb

X-ray beam centering
- direct vertical beam at the patella
- proximodistal beam is directed 10° craniocaudally to project the joint surfaces more completely

Collimation
- include patella and femoropatellar joint

Comments

- dog is bearing weight on the tibia of the affected limb, with the quadriceps tendon pulled tightly
- it may be stressful and painful to position the limb in this manner
- palpate the patella to determine the specific angle of the X-ray beam thought best to evaluate the joint spaces
- decrease radiographic technique because of minimal tissue thickness

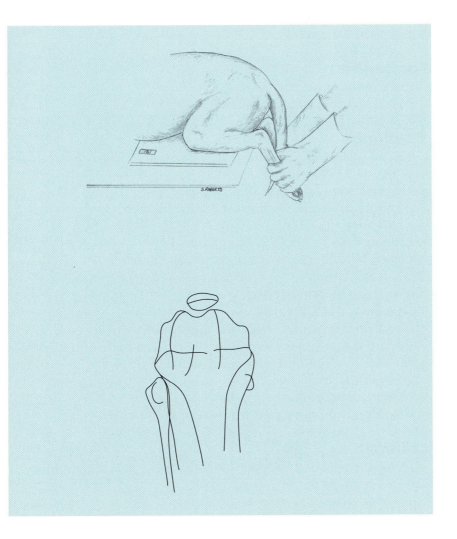

Patella – caudocranial view with horizontal beam

Body
- place in lateral recumbency on pad, with affected limb uppermost
- use compression band over thorax

Head and neck
- place head in neutral position
- place sandbag over neck

Forelimbs
- place limbs in neutral position
- place sandbags across forelimbs

Hindlimbs
- extend unaffected limb in neutral position
  - place sandbag on limb
- elevate affected limb on sponge block
- position cassette vertically just cranial to stifle
- tightly flex stifle joint
- use sandbags to hold cassette against limb
- hold limb using sandbags or use gloved hand

X-ray beam centering
- reposition the X-ray tube caudally
- direct the horizontal beam in a caudocranial direction
- palpate the patella to determine the correct angle of the beam
- the angle of the beam is approximately 90° to the longitudinal axis of the femur
- center the beam on the patella
- the beam need not be perpendicular to the cassette

Collimation
- include patella and femoropatellar joint

Comments

- this view provides a good study of the patella but requires extensive repositioning of the X-ray tube
- the technique is relatively painless because the dog does not bear weight on the patella or stifle joint
- incomplete flexion of the stifle in the injured patient may limit the effectiveness of the view

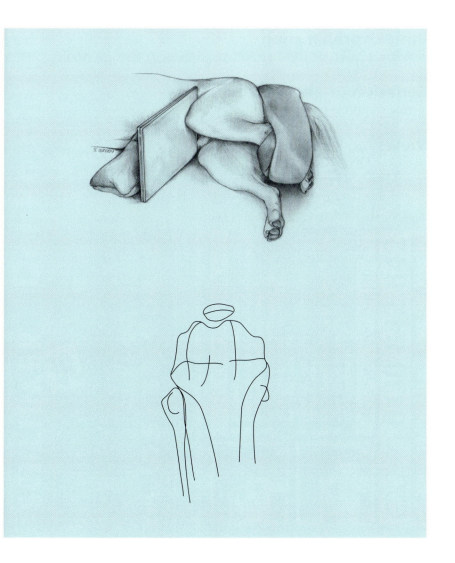

Tibia and Fibula

Introduction
– examinations of the tibia and fibula usually follow trauma
– these bones are relatively easy to radiograph because they are distal in the limb and have only a minimal amount of soft tissue surrounding them

Patient preparation
– inspect haircoat for matted hair, debris, or foreign bodies

Sedation or anesthesia
– not required for all views

Views
– recommended views
  – lateral view
  – caudocranial view using vertical beam
– special views
  – oblique views

X-ray technique
– medium to low kVp may permit better evaluation of bone

Use of grid
– studies do not require use of a grid

Comments
– views of the opposite limb need to be made in puppies up to 9 to 12 months to permit comparison of growth centers

Tibia and fibula – lateral view

Body
- place in lateral recumbency on side to be studied
- use a compression band over thorax

Head and neck
- place head in neutral position
- place sandbag over neck

Forelimbs
- place limbs in neutral position
- hold limbs with sandbags

Hindlimbs
- unaffected limb is either flexed, extended, or abducted and removed from radiation field
- place cassette on table top
- place affected limb on cassette
- partially extend affected limb with stifle partially flexed
- hold limb with sandbag over foot and femur or use tie-down rope or use gloved hand

X-ray beam centering
- direct vertical beam on midshaft of tibia

Collimation
- include stifle, tibia and fibula, and talocrural joint

Comments

– this is a relatively easy view to make

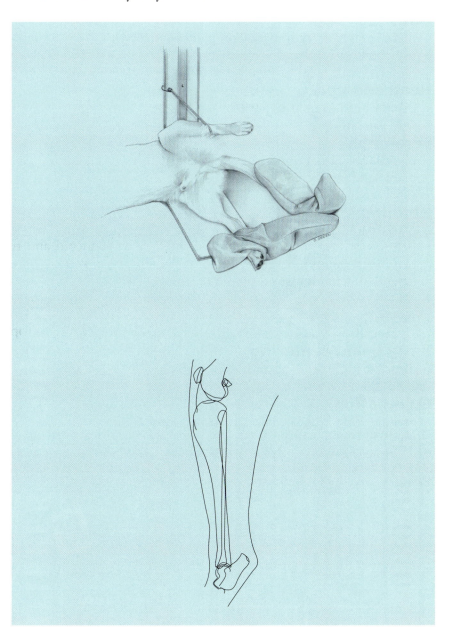

Tibia and fibula – caudocranial view

Body
– place in sternal recumbency on pad or in trough
– use compression band across back

Head and neck
– extend head in neutral position

Forelimbs
– place limbs in neutral position
– place sandbags across limbs

Hindlimbs
– place unaffected limb on sponge block to elevate limb and rotate pelvis
– place cassette on table top
– extend affected limb and place on cassette
– place sandbags across feet or use tie-down rope or use gloved hand

X-ray beam centering
– direct vertical beam at midshaft of tibia

Collimation
– include stifle, tibia and fibula, and talocrural joint

Comments

– avoid axial rotation of the limb
– may be less painful if a sponge is placed under the patella of the affected limb

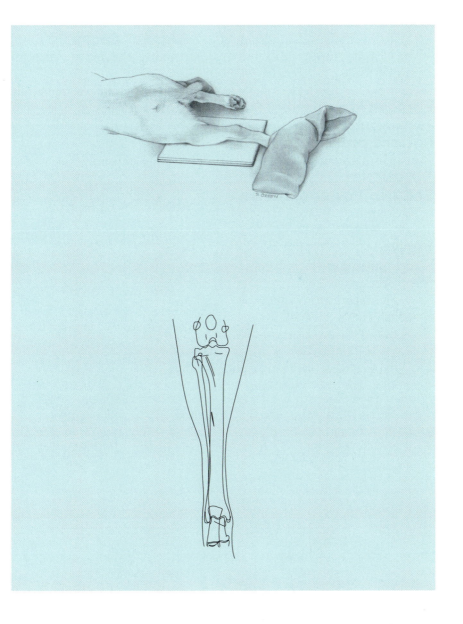

Tarsus, Metatarsus, and Digits

Introduction
- examinations of the feet are relatively easy to perform because of the ease in positioning and only minimal soft tissue thickness
- the techniques are similar in radiography of all parts of the foot
- stress radiography is useful in determining the extent of joint injury
- use positioning devices such as a wooden spoon or plastic paddle to assist in positioning of the foot for stress studies

Patient preparation
- inspect haircoat for matted hair, debris, or foreign bodies

Sedation or anesthesia
- not required for most studies

Views
- recommended views
  - lateral view
  - plantarodorsal view
- special views
  - oblique views
  - dorsoplantar view with foot stressed
  - hyperflexed or hyperextended views

X-ray technique
– medium to low kVp may permit better evaluation of bone

Use of grid
– studies are performed using a table top method without a grid

Comments
– views of the opposite limb are recommended in puppies up to 9
  to 12 months of age so that the appearance of growth centers can
  be compared in both limbs

Tarsus, metatarsus, and digits – lateral view

Body
- place in lateral recumbency on side to be studied
- use a compression band over thorax

Head and neck
- place head in neutral position
- place sandbag over neck

Forelimbs
- place limb in a neutral position
- place sandbags over limbs

Hindlimbs
- remove upper limb from field by caudal displacement
- hold limb with tie-down rope or sandbag
- position the affected limb cranially extended
- place cassette on table top
- position foot on cassette in neutral, hyperflexed, or hyperextended position
- hold limb with sandbag or tie-down rope or positioning device

X-ray beam centering
- direct vertical beam on the foot

Collimation
- include distal tibia and fibula, talocrural joint, tarsus, metatarsus, and digits

Comments
- hold foot in 90° flexion with tibia for neutral study
- use positioning device to create hyperextension or hyperflexion stress studies
- can hold positioning device with sandbag
- it is helpful to reposition a digit using a gauze strip to force a hyperextended position so that the digit is not covered by the other digits

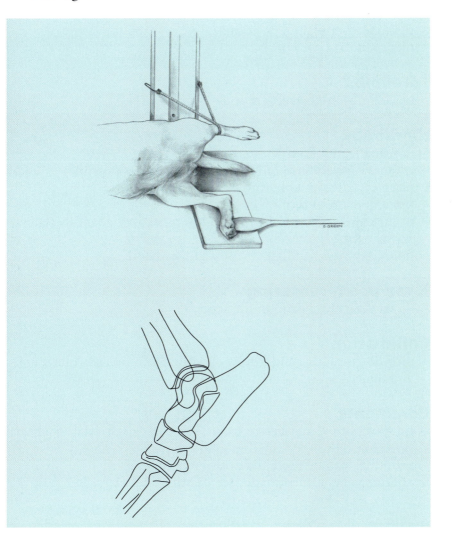

Tarsus, metatarsus, and digits – plantarodorsal view

Body
- place in sternal recumbency on pad or in trough
- use compression band across back

Head and neck
- place head in neutral position
- place sandbag over neck

Forelimbs
- place limbs in neutral position

Hindlimbs
- flex unaffected limb
- extend affected limb caudally as completely as possible
- place cassette on table top
- place dorsum of foot on cassette
- position neutrally, axially (medially) stressed, or abaxially (laterally) stressed
- hold limb with sandbag or use a gloved hand

X-ray beam centering
- direct a vertical beam on the foot

Collimation
- include distal tibia and fibula, talocrural joint, tarsus, metatarsus, and digits

Comments
- use positioning devices to create pressure in an axial or abaxial direction
- a sandbag can be used as a positioning device
- oblique views can be made (see drawings below)

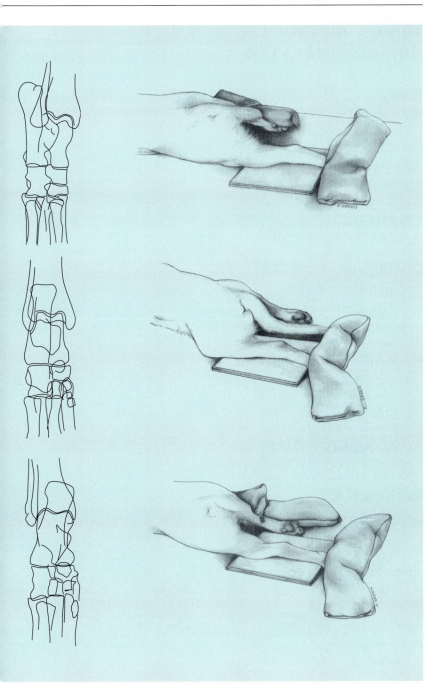

Tarsus, metatarsus, and digits – dorsoplantar view

Body
– position dog sitting on table top

Head and neck
– place head in neutral position
– place sandbag over neck

Forelimbs
– supported by assistant

Hindlimbs
– flex unaffected limb
– extend affected limb cranially as completely as possible by placing hand pressure on the stifle joint
– place cassette on table top
– place foot on cassette
– position neutrally, axially (medially) stressed, or abaxially (laterally) stressed
– hold limb with gloved hand

X-ray beam centering
– direct a vertical beam on the foot

Collimation
– include distal tibia and fibula, talocrural joint, tarsus, metatarsus, and digits

Comments

- use positioning devices to create pressure in an axial or abaxial direction
- can use sandbag to hold positioning device
- foot can be rotated internally or externally to permit oblique views of the foot
- use a plastic paddle to force the foot against the cassette to prevent flexion of the digits

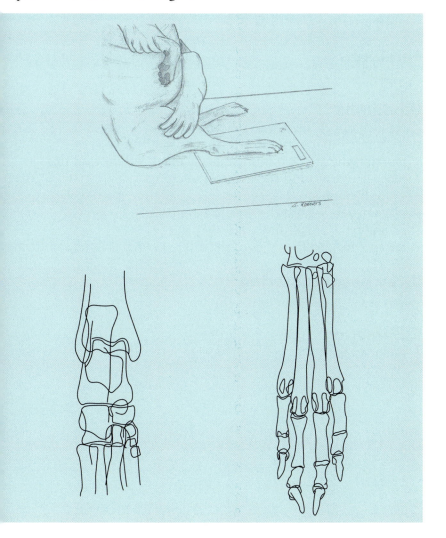

Digits – lateral view

Body
- place in lateral recumbency on side to be studied
- place a compression band over abdomen

Head and neck
- place head in neutral position
- place sandbag over neck

Forelimbs
- place sandbags over limbs

Hindlimbs
- remove upper limb from field by flexion
  - hold limb with tie-down rope or sandbag
- position the affected limb cranially extended on cassette
- place gauze around the unaffected digits
  - pull in a plantar direction
- place gauze around the affected digit
  - pull in a dorsal direction
- fasten gauze to the edge of the table or wrap around sandbags

X-ray beam centering
- direct vertical beam on the digits

Collimation
- include digits

Comments
– the affected digit is separated by pulling on both gauze strips

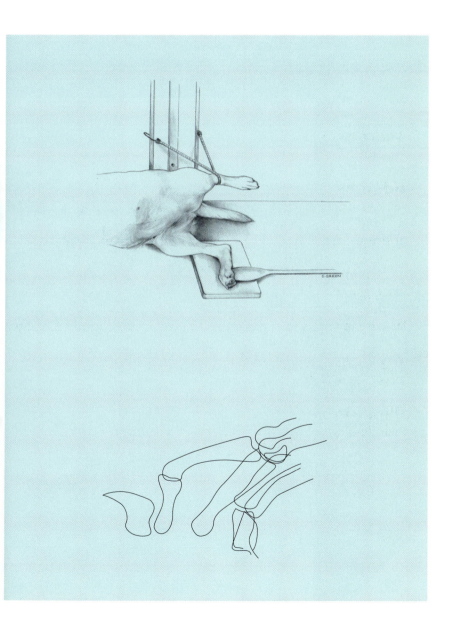

Notes